SECRETS

of the

ICEWOMEN

The Power *of*
Cold *and* Breathwork
to Balance Hormones,
Bolster Health, *and* Unlock
Inner Potential

SECRETS

of the

ICEWOMEN

ISABELLE HOF and LAURA HOF

HARPER

An Imprint of HarperCollinsPublishers

SECRETS OF THE ICEWOMEN. Copyright © 2025 by Isabelle Hof and Laura Hof. All rights reserved. Printed in the United States of America. No part of this book may be used or reproduced in any manner whatsoever without written permission except in the case of brief quotations embodied in critical articles and reviews. For information, address HarperCollins Publishers, 195 Broadway, New York, NY 10007.

HarperCollins books may be purchased for educational, business, or sales promotional use. For information, please email the Special Markets Department at SPsales@harpercollins.com.

FIRST EDITION

Library of Congress Cataloging-in-Publication Data has been applied for.

ISBN 978-0-06-339160-4

25 26 27 28 29 LBC 5 4 3 2 1

We want to dedicate this book to our mother.
Without the journey and the lessons learned from her passing,
this book would never exist.

CONTENTS

INTRODUCTION

On a cold winter morning in 2020, Storm Dennis was in full force, sweeping over the Netherlands. While many chose to stay cozy indoors, wrapped in warm clothes and woolen socks, we had other plans. It was barely nine a.m., and, surrounded by sheets of rain and howling wind, we took our very first dip with the newly founded Icewomen Community, a group we started to empower more women to experience the unique-to-women benefits of cold water dipping. In Dutch, we have a saying: "Weather or no weather," which means that no matter what's going on outside, we keep going. And that's what we did!

Somehow, the discomfort of that day—with the storm wreaking havoc around us—allowed the cold to bring us even more serenity. Surrounded by other strong, resilient women, we became the eye of the storm. From that day on, the winter and autumn seasons became our favorite time to come together. Our gatherings are always filled with positivity, serenity, and of course, a sense of accomplishment and excitement afterward. Since that day, the Icewomen Community has grown not just in the Netherlands but across the world—from the US to Spain to Guatemala—as more women began gathering to unite in their shared love of the cold.

It's the thousands of women entering our Wim Hof Method (WHM) workshops, travels, retreats, and Icewomen gatherings, and even becoming WHM instructors, whom we first want to thank, because all of the questions they asked over the years showed us this book was necessary. Questions like: *Where do I find more information about the method and female-specific health conditions? Can I use the method to support me through menstrual cycles, pregnancy, or menopause? Do breathwork and the cold affect women and men differently?*

So many great questions! We have tried to answer as many as we could over the years, sharing anecdotes and observations while we continue to push more research on the impacts of the WHM on women specifically. Now, this book gives us a chance to address all of the questions in one place, and to give the women in our community and beyond a place to start establishing a female-centered approach to the method.

This book contains information about the WHM in relation to women, and we share tips and techniques that are especially important for women. Women face an incredible burden of stress, and our hormones fluctuate each month and throughout our lives, affecting our bodies, physiology, and even brain structure. These changes influence our body temperature regulation, how warm or cold we feel, and our breathing rhythms. This makes it not just beneficial but critical to approach women's health and wellness, and the way they practice the WHM—with an approach that addresses the mysterious and incredible variation within us.

In this book we'll dive deep into female physiology and the three pillars of the WHM—cold, breath, and mindset—before getting into the specific benefits that the WHM offers for women, as we've seen through both research and our firsthand experience. Then, we'll take you through a 30-Day Icewoman Challenge to introduce you to the WHM in a way that is digestible, manageable, and easy to implement at home. To deepen your understanding of the exact practice of the Wim Hof Method, we always recommend a WHM workshop.

Before we dive in, a word on safety. Challenging yourself is a fundamental part of the Wim Hof Method, but it's important to know your limits and always prioritize safety. Always practice the WHM breathing exercises sitting or lying down in a safe environment. The Wim Hof Method breathing can affect motor control and, in rare cases, lead to loss of consciousness. This is why we always communicate to never practice while driving, in or near water, or in any place where loss of consciousness could lead to bodily harm. For those who have never done any form of cold exposure, always remember to *gradually build up*. The cold is a powerful force and can be a shock to your body if you're not properly prepared and trained. Avoid practicing the method during pregnancy or if you have epilepsy. People with cardiovascular health issues, or any other serious health conditions, should always consult with a medical doctor before starting the Wim Hof Method. Always listen to your body and never force the practice.

Our hope is that this book lands in the hands of every woman practicing the Wim Hof Method, and that it helps them align with the deepest parts of themselves, and makes them feel whole. If you are holding this book right now, we hope it magnifies your strength and shifts your energy. We hope it helps you break through societal conditioning, external expectations, and fear. We hope it helps you create balance and peace within, so you have more peace in your life. We strongly believe that the WHM is one of the most potent natural tools you can have in your backpack to go on this human journey we call life, giving you more sovereignty over your own happiness, health, and strength. The shiver-inducing pictures of people in ice baths or frozen lakes can often alienate women, holding them back from its life-changing effects. The wall between women and the WHM is already crumbling, and our hope is that this book will kick it all the way down—officially inviting every woman in.

SECRETS

of the

ICEWOMEN

1

THE WIM HOF METHOD

"The impossible is possible."

The Wim Hof Method (WHM) today involves online courses, facilities, workshops, and retreats all over the world with highly trained instructors. But all of this only became part of the picture recently. Before the WHM that you know today, our dad was known as more of an extreme outlier, a crazy stunt guy who attracted a lot of attention for his many superhuman feats—he climbed Mount Everest in shorts, ran a half marathon above the Arctic Circle barefoot, and stood in a container while covered with ice cubes for more than 112 minutes. It took him more than four decades to go from being seen as a circus act to being a respected figure in health and medicine.

This scientific interest was key to the development of the Wim Hof Method as we know it today. Science is the primary means by which we acquire knowledge about the natural world. Through systematic observation, experimentation, and analysis, the fundamental principles and laws that govern our universe are uncovered.

This knowledge forms the foundation for our understanding of the things around us and helps us navigate this complex world. Without the interest of scientists, our dad, Wim Hof, might have simply remained a human anomaly who was capable of extreme feats. Thanks to science, we now know why our father was able to withstand the cold for so long, and we know that all of us can benefit from his practices, too.

FROM ICEMAN TO THE WIM HOF METHOD

Our dad's relationship with science and healthcare started in 2007, when he flew to the United States to set a new Guinness World Record. He broke the record, sitting in an ice bucket in the middle of Times Square in New York for two hours, sixteen minutes, and thirty-four seconds. On the same trip, he also went to the Feinstein Institutes for Medical Research so they could run some medical tests on him. Dr. Kevin Tracey, the president and CEO of the Feinstein Institutes for Medical Research and famous for his study of the nervous system, was interested in Wim's ability to endure the cold. Dr. Tracey was especially interested in observing Wim's autonomic nervous system, which regulates involuntary processes like heart rate, blood pressure, respiration, digestion, and sexual arousal. They hooked our dad up to some machines while he did meditation and breathing exercises, and then tested his blood for 307 different biomarkers. The results showed evidence that Wim Hof could influence the behavior of his autonomic nervous system, which was thought to be impossible at that time. In a letter outlining the results of the study, Dr. Tracey suggested that Wim Hof's meditation and breathing techniques gave him the capability to effectively stimulate the vagus nerve, which is instrumental for getting us to a state of relaxation and restoration, and that we may all have that innate potential.

In 2009, while our father was setting another world record—for sitting in a bucket of ice up to the neck wearing only shorts—another researcher was collecting data on him. Wim was asked to swallow a Vital Sense monitor capsule that would capture his core body temperature while he was in the ice bucket. This was done in partnership with Dr. Ken Kamler, a physician who has practiced medicine in some of the most extreme conditions on Earth, including Antarctica, and worked as the chief high-altitude physician for NASA. During this experiment, Dr. Kamler's team observed our dad's core body temperature drop all the way to 87.9°F and then increase again to 97.52°F without any external source of heat. This showed his incredible control over his own physiology. As Dr. Kamler wrote in a follow-up letter:

> Standard medical dogma states that once your core temperature falls below 35°C/90°F you stop shivering... from that point on, if a source of external heat is not provided, your body temperature will continue to spiral downward, and you will eventually die of hypothermia. Wim has proven this wrong. . . . He has dramatically shown us that there is incredible power within the human body that modern medicine does not clearly understand.

Wim Hof defied medical theory and showed, once again, that the impossible is possible. Dr. Kamler told our dad that if he could reproduce these results, it would mean huge consequences for humankind and open a whole new era of research into the nervous system. This was the moment our father's true mission began—to show the world not just what he could do, but that he could teach others to do it, too.

The next scientist to enter the picture was Dr. Marianne Hopman, a professor of physiology at Radboud University Medical Center who studies chronic diseases and their underlying mechanisms. She became interested in studying our father because of the early observations that he could consciously influence his autonomic nervous system. In 2010 and 2011, Dr. Hopman conducted three experiments measuring our dad's inflammatory response while practicing the WHM. He was injected with pieces of dead *E. coli* bacteria, and his immune response was compared to that of 112 other people who had also been injected. All the other participants showed symptoms of immune activation, like fever and fatigue. But our father didn't get sick after being injected. His blood showed lower inflammatory proteins, and even after a period of six days, he had a higher white blood cell count than the other participants. This study laid the foundation for studying Wim Hof's abilities and protocols in the context of not just the nervous system but immune health, which led directly to the most famous study on Wim—the 2014 Radboud study.

THE 2014 RADBOUD STUDY

In science, an experiment on one person is called a "case study." And while it can reveal incredible information, like the 2012 study on our father did, it only holds so much weight. It may show amazing results, but it does not prove that the results are directly applicable to others. Scientists had observed that Wim Hof was capable of incredible things, but was he the only one? Or could others be trained in our dad's techniques and see the same results for themselves? Radboud University was eager to find out. They partnered with our father to conduct a now-famous 2014 study called "Voluntary Activation of the Sympathetic Nervous System and Attenuation of the Innate Immune Response in Humans." For this study, Wim Hof trained eighteen men, from whom twelve were randomly selected to participate in the experiment, and then compared them to a control group undergoing various immune and nervous system tests.

Isabelle: I remember when I first heard about the Radboud study. My dad and I were in the Netherlands driving around, and he was telling me that he was in conversation with Radboud about the number of days he would have to train the eighteen people. I wondered if he would say years, months, or weeks, so I was surprised when my dad said confidently that ten days would be enough! Shocked, I looked at him with blank eyes and said: "But you are so experienced and well trained, do you really think you can do this in ten days? What if that's not enough time to train them?" I was thinking to myself that it can take years for the body to adapt, and he wants to teach this group of participants in just ten days to do something that has never been done by anyone but Wim himself? It could jeopardize the whole effort to show the capabilities of the method. But my dad was steadfast, adamant that ten days would do. Needless to say, I was biting my nails. Looking back, I now realize that a big part of our dad's method is to have belief!

Surrounded by researchers, Wim Hof took the eighteen men on a four-day training in Poland. They practiced Wim's breathing and mindset exercises and immersed themselves in ice water. He even took them on a snowy climb in the Karkonoska mountain pass on the Polish-Czech border in their shorts. He knew the group of men were ready when they did the Harlem Shake, dancing on top of the mountain! Back in the Netherlands, they trained independently for six more days, priming their mindset and practicing cold exposure and daily breathing exercises. Immediately after the training, twelve out of the eighteen participants were injected with *E. coli* in the hospital and observed.

The results were remarkable. The participants who were not trained by Wim Hof fell sick with nausea, headaches, shivers, and fevers just as expected. In contrast, 100 percent of the participants in the WHM group felt completely fine and had no or minor symptoms. The contrast was striking. The results showed that, like our father, they were also able to influence their autonomic nervous system and immune system. The trained group's anti-inflammatory mediators were a whopping 200 percent higher, their pro-inflammatory mediators were 50 percent lower, and they had significantly more white blood cells, which had important implications for people suffering from conditions involving inflammation and the immune system.

WHAT IS INFLAMMATION? Inflammation is a normal, healthy response of the body that occurs when we have an infection or injury. All of us will experience inflammation in our lives; for example, when our ankle swells and gets red after an injury, or when we develop mucus and a fever when we're fighting an infection. Our bodies sense a threat, and they respond by releasing chemicals in the body that cause inflammation to protect us. So, when does the problem with inflammation occur? It happens when our inflammation becomes constant—known as chronic inflammation—and our body doesn't have a chance to recover and clean up after inflammation is triggered. Having long-term low-grade inflammation in the body eventually seems to deregulate the immune system and can lead to a wide range of diseases.

The results of this study were published in 2014 in the renowned journal *PNAS* (*Proceedings of the National Academy of Sciences of the United States of America*), which established more credibility for Wim's techniques and further piqued the interest of scientists. This study is what really kicked off mainstream interest in the method and gave it a scientific backbone.

WHERE'S ALL THE RESEARCH ON WOMEN? You may have noticed that the first few studies on the WHM were on men only. This is a symptom of a much larger problem. Overall, women are studied in medical research far less often, with only 28 percent of studies including women in 2009. Instead, women were just considered "smaller men" and excluded from clinical trials because of concerns that their monthly hormone fluctuations would disrupt results. The consequences of this have been dire for women. For example, researchers from the University of Chicago analyzed studies in which women were given the same drug dosage as men and found that in 90 percent of cases, women experienced stronger side effects than men and experienced adverse drug reactions at nearly twice the rate of men. This has changed some in recent years, as the number of studies that included females grew to 49 percent in 2019. But in eight of the nine fields studied, the proportion that analyzed results by sex did not improve. In pharmacology, the trend of women being included in studies spiraled downward, from 33 percent to 29 percent. This is one of the reasons why Dr. Elissa Epel, professor of psychiatry at the University of California San Francisco (UCSF), was interested in studying the effect of WHM on stress, mood, and depression in women specifically. This study is in the process of being published but preliminary results showed that the WHM improved stress in women, leading to significantly more daily positive emotions, with long-term benefits.

The study revealed for the first time in history that we all *can* influence our autonomic nervous system and our immune system at will—something that was previously thought of as impossible. Before this study, every textbook stated we cannot influence our autonomic nervous system, and every doctor was taught the same in school.

The gravity of this scientific breakthrough meant that we needed to rethink what humans are capable of. It was a real paradigm shift.

As Peter Pickkers, professor of experimental intensive care at Radboud Medical University, said: "That a human being can willfully influence their autonomic nervous system, has now been proven scientifically without a doubt. This was the first time in history. It has never been done before." In his hospital bed, surrounded by doctors, professors, and researchers, our father was asked by an interviewer from a Dutch news outlet if the experiment was hard to go through, and his answer revealed a lot about his inner world throughout his journey:

> For me it was easy. You know what was hard? The road leading up to this, to show that this is possible. The mockery, the assaults, the unbelief. . . . When this is all over . . . I will cry.

We remember when these results were published, and how the news of this paradigm shift didn't spread right away. In fact, it might have been entirely off the radar if it wasn't for the endless devotion and enthusiasm of our dad. It took some time for local newspapers and TV to cover it, and eventually it spread internationally. Our dad's voice finally grew louder through international podcasts like those of Tim Ferriss and Joe Rogan and a beautiful documentary on VICE. On any given day, he would work hard and push this message forward, spreading his techniques to anybody who was interested (and sometimes even to those who were not that interested). Our dad is always extremely passionate and enthusiastic during podcasts and documentaries for large audiences; he is equally passionate talking with taxi drivers, nurses, and anyone else who he thinks could benefit from the method. He was always sure that his ability to influence the autonomic nervous system was something everybody could do with some training, and now it was backed by science. He managed to reach and connect with audiences big and small. Like all his other accomplishments, he was relentless in his pursuit to spread awareness of the method.

The 2014 Radboud study was groundbreaking, and more research quickly followed. A number of studies into the WHM pertaining to the autonomic nervous system, immune system, stress levels, and even specific ailments and diseases were published in the coming years, shedding more light on the "magic" behind Wim Hof's abilities. The results of these studies deepened our understanding of the method and its possible applications in mainstream healthcare, and we outline many of them in this very book when we dive into the benefits of the Wim Hof Method. This early research also led to our father developing the Wim Hof Method, which defined the three pillars behind the practice he'd developed over decades and allowed others to learn.

THE 3 PILLARS OF THE WHM

The Wim Hof Method is divided into three pillars: cold, breath, and mindset. By combining cold exposure, breathing techniques, and the power of the mind we reignite the full potential of our physiology. As a result, we gain much more control over not just our health but our happiness. With the Wim Hof Method, we rebalance our nervous system, boost our immune system, and create mental resilience.

Pillar 1: Cold Exposure

The first pillar of the Wim Hof Method is cold exposure. The cold is an extreme force that activates the most primal parts of our brain. When we go into the cold, we stop thinking about anything else and break the stream of continuous thought in our heads, anchoring us in the "here and now." Our 30-plus trillion cells respond to this short-term intense stressor by activating our adaptive mechanisms. They reshape the internal landscape of our bodies to prepare for the next bout of stress, making us more resilient on a cellular level.

When we get into the cold, we:

- Train our cardiovascular system and lymphatic system
- Learn to deal with stress
- Increase focus and mental capacity
- Activate "feel-good" hormones
- Produce cold shock proteins with longevity benefits
- Activate stem cells
- Improve sleep
- Optimize our metabolism
- Activate our brown fat and increase cell metabolic activity
- Detox our bodies
- Lower inflammation
- Increase the production of white blood cells
- Increase production of growth hormone in the brain

This pillar also makes us more physically, emotionally, and mentally resilient. When we do something uncomfortable, we learn to take back the reins over our stress response. After all, the stress response telling us to get out of the ice is the same one that's at play when our boss calls, when we're arguing with our spouse, when we're stuck in traffic, when we're worried about money, or when our children are screaming and kicking. If we complete the practice, our bodies reward us by flooding us with happy hormones. We feel happier, stronger, and healthier, and benefit from a sharper mind and increased confidence.

Pillar 2: Breathing

The Wim Hof Method involves various breathing techniques that play with the chemistry of our bodies, leading to a cascade of health benefits. We have different techniques for different purposes, but in our workshops and classes, we teach you the WHM Basic Breathing exercise, which was the exercise used in most scientific research. With the basic WHM breathing exercise, we alternate between phases of deep active breathing and moments where we pause our breathing mindfully (called breath holds or breath retention).

These breathing exercises act as a full respiratory system workout. In return, the body sets up a cascade of protective mechanisms that change and strengthen our physiology. We use our breath to:

- Energize the body and increase metabolism
- Train the cardiovascular system and the lungs
- Massage the tissues and muscles around the lungs and the diaphragm
- Increase blood circulation
- Reduce inflammation and improve the immune response system
- Lower stress and reset the nervous system
- Increase pain tolerance
- Become more resilient toward the cold
- Tap into our emotions and deal with trauma
- Become more oxygen-efficient and CO_2 tolerant
- Enter a meditative state of being
- Regulate our mental and emotional state

When we tell people who have never experimented with the breath what it can do, they often respond with disbelief. We literally "get high on our own supply." People report kaleidoscopic visuals, out-of-body experiences, seeing other dimensions, healing from past trauma by witnessing past experiences from a different lens, and even talking to their ancestors or family members (both deceased and alive!). These altered states of consciousness are accessible within a fifteen-to-twenty-minute breathing session. We'll talk more about these amazing benefits in Chapter 5, but this is a glimpse of how powerful the breathing exercises can be.

With the WHM breathing exercise, we acquire the abilities of advanced yogis or monks. We go to realms that you only read about in books, but without training for decades or giving up our worldly possessions. We can take advantage of these benefits as real people with ups and downs, busy schedules and families, jobs, and kids.

Pillar 3: Mindset

The final pillar is all about the mind. This third piece of the puzzle is often overlooked, since both breathwork and cold immersion are tangible things you can see, hear, and touch. Mindset is often more difficult to understand before you experience it, but it's truly the cornerstone of the Wim Hof Method. As you've read, in many of the studies on Wim, he was able to influence his autonomic nervous system through sheer force of will. Wim showed that by rehearsing and visualizing a situation using his mind, he could have his body react as though it were real.

At its core, the WHM is about cultivating a powerful mindset, and we do this by strengthening the mind-body connection. Like training a muscle in the gym, we build the muscle that connects the body and the mind. Just like focus can be trained, through meditation, we can also learn to use the mind. Belief is a powerful tool, and if we exercise it, we can make new neural connections and see real, tangible benefits. Learn to use your mind, and it will become your best friend, enabling you to make the impossible possible.

With the Wim Hof Method, you learn how to use the power of your mind. As our father likes to say: "The sky is not the limit; the limit is the mind."

The pillars separately are already extremely powerful, but scientific research shows that the combination of the pillars is the strongest. All three pillars conspire to create the benefits behind the WHM.

It's not always easy to turn the shower to cold or hop into an ice bath, but with each attempt, we fortify our mental muscles and learn to deal with discomfort, gaining confidence that guides us in the next round of cold exposure or through the next challenge in life.

FROM ICEMAN TO ICEWOMEN

When we talk about the history behind the Wim Hof Method, we can't ignore the elephant in the room: since its inception, the WHM was dominated by men. When we first started teaching workshops and trainings, at least 80 percent of the participants were men. In fact, it was a special treat for a woman to be in one of our workshops or activities, and we used to joke that if you were a straight single lady, it would be the best place to find a date!

We suspect there were more men than women at first because Wim was the face of the method. After all, he really does look like a wintry caveman. The ice baths can seem harsh or overly extreme for many women. But slowly, this has started to change. First, it was just a woman every few sessions, but then that woman would invite her friend or sister, who would then invite her coworker, mom, or childhood friend until our trainings started looking a lot different. These days our trainings are about 35 to 40 percent women, and we hold women-only retreats. Women have become the backbone of our community.

As we have observed more and more women try the WHM, what has really struck us is just how profound the benefits for women seem to be. Increasingly, women were not just trying the WHM, they were completely transforming their lives with it. We believe this has everything to do with the WHM's ability to counteract the effects of chronic stress so many women are under. It's no surprise to us that there was a drastic increase in female WHM practitioners during the COVID pandemic, as many women were burdened by even more stress than usual—struggling to manage parenting, work, life, and relationships. In the next chapter, we'll dive into the intricate physiology of the nervous system, the epidemic of chronic stress among women, and how the WHM may be the solution so many women desperately need.

WOMEN AND THE STRESS OF A MAN'S WORLD

"Bless the stress."

The WHM affects our nervous system on a fundamental level, allowing us to build a foundation of resiliency and calm. As we'll learn in this chapter, managing chronic stress is absolutely critical for women all over the world to achieve health and happiness. Women are more likely to suffer from chronic stress—and the health conditions caused by it—due to historical, cultural, societal, and neurobiological reasons.

The WHM gives women an avenue to learn about the physiology of stress and how it's affecting their lives, and provides them the tools they need to thrive.

MOTHER NATURE'S RHYTHM AND OUR MODERN LIFESTYLE

Our human physiology is a product of millions of years of evolution, perfected to be symbiotic to the natural rhythms of the Earth.

For example, our bodies adapt to the seasons and the differences in temperature and light throughout the year. We move in harmony with the cycle of each day, releasing the hormone cortisol in the morning in response to sunlight and the sleep hormone melatonin in the evening in response to lack of light in our environment.

For women, we even deal with additional natural cycles, such as the monthly cycle, the pregnancy cycle, and the menopause cycle. These cycles last longer than the twenty-four-hour circadian rhythm and are called infradian rhythms. Women's bodies, just like the planets, the sun, and the moon, cycle naturally and assume different rhythms at different phases. It's clear when we look at the way a woman's body works that we are constantly adapting to fluctuations in our internal and external environment, which means there are many more opportunities for our bodies to get out of sync.

Our autonomic nervous system is a critical piece of the puzzle when it comes to being in tune with our environments. You can think of it as the bridge between the external world and our inner ecosystem. Its main objective is to keep our internal ecosystem balanced so we can thrive; which means regulating things like body temperature, heart rate, breathing, sweat production, and the immune system, which all need to be stable and within a very specific range. This balance is called homeostasis, a term derived from the Greek word for "same" and "steady." Our bodies are constantly working to keep this homeostatic balance in check through something called neuroception, a phenomenon where the nervous system constantly scans for cues of safety or danger without using the conscious, "thinking" parts of the brain. This means we are mostly unaware of this happening behind the scenes every minute of the day, but the nervous system constantly responds and recalibrates in response to the environment, pushing toward homeostasis.

Anything that threatens this homeostatic balance can be defined as "stress," and the automatic reaction toward perceived or real threats (stressors) is called the "stress response." Most of us take this part of our physiology for granted, but the truth is the processing capacity of our subconscious brains is two hundred thousand times larger than the conscious part. This part of our brain can process 11.2 million bits per second, where the conscious can process, at maximum, only 60 bits per second.

HOMEOSTASIS VS. ALLOSTASIS: "Homeostasis" refers to the body's ability to maintain a stable internal environment despite external changes. It involves processes that keep physiological parameters like temperature, pH, and fluid balance within a narrow, optimal range. For example, when you're exposed to cold temperatures, your body shivers to generate heat and maintain a stable core temperature. "Allostasis," on the other hand, refers to the process of achieving stability through change. It's a more dynamic concept that involves the body's ability to adapt to stressors and changing conditions over time. Allostasis considers that the body might need to adjust its normal ranges to deal with new or prolonged stressors, like adapting to extreme cold. Repeated exposure to cold through WHM training can lead to long-term adaptations. Your body may become more efficient at managing cold stress, such as improving circulation, enhancing metabolic rate, and increasing tolerance to cold. This ongoing adaptation is an example of allostasis, where the body adjusts its stress response systems to handle cold exposure better over time.

The nervous system is an amazing mechanism, designed to keep us safe from threats to our life and health. But here's the challenge: Our stress response was designed when humans' lives were very different from those we live today. Gone are the days that we must flee quickly from a hungry lion or chase an animal down for our next meal. Today, we are not dealing with very many real dangers like we had to deal with as cavewomen. Instead, we experience constant low-grade stress on our brain and body, including:

- Work stress, such as burnout, job anxiety, long hours
- Dietary stressors, such as a high-sugar, low-nutrient diet, and alcohol use
- Physical stressors, such as a sedentary lifestyle or medication use
- Societal stressors, such as politics, violence, crime, and war
- Environmental stressors, like toxins and climate change
- Economic stressors, such as recession
- Health stressors, such as chronic disease or being a caretaker

Our nervous systems have not adapted to understand that these stressors are not hungry lions to run from, which leads to a constant and elevated activation of the nervous system.

THE SYMPATHETIC NERVOUS SYSTEM: FIGHT-FLIGHT-FREEZE

The autonomic nervous system can be further broken down into two branches: the sympathetic nervous system (SNS) and the parasympathetic nervous system (PNS). These two branches work together like the gas and the brake pedals, with our SNS responsible for our "fight, flight, or freeze" response and our PNS responsible for our "rest and digest" response. When it comes to the SNS, you can further break it down into short-term and long-term activation.

The Stress Response: The Short Version

Imagine you come home from a long day at work and put your coat and bag in the hallway. After a quick stop at the bathroom, you head to the kitchen for tea and snacks. You settle on the couch, close your eyes briefly, then hear a noise upstairs. A shock runs through you—was that real? Then you hear it again, followed by footsteps. Your body goes into fight-or-flight mode. Your mind races. Should you scream, call the police, or run? You may freeze, overwhelmed by thoughts, emotions, and a pounding heart—all triggered by your sympathetic nervous system.

When a stressor is first perceived (in this case, the footsteps upstairs), the activation of the sympathetic nervous system leads to the release of adrenaline and noradrenaline into the bloodstream. These hormones prepare the body for immediate action, triggering important changes in the body. Your heart starts to pump faster, your blood pressure goes up, your airways dilate to absorb more oxygen, and your brain, heart, lungs, and essential muscles receive more blood. Adrenaline also speeds up metabolism and releases glucose into the bloodstream for extra energy. This response temporarily inhibits nonessential functions, such as digestion and reproductive processes, to redirect energy where it's most needed. This reaction is called your fight-flight-freeze response. Your body is getting ready to fight for its life, hide in total silence, or run. The world shifts sharply into focus, time slows down, and our reactions quicken and become razor-sharp.

But then, just when you decide to run out of the house and call the police, you realize that the person upstairs is your daughter. You take a deep breath and start walking upstairs. Your heart rate quickly goes back to normal, and you feel the tension in your body ease. This is the other branch of your autonomic nervous system, called your parasympathetic nervous system (PNS), taking over. You give your child a long, tight hug. The parasympathetic system activates when we feel safe and gives us a feeling of calm and promotes a state of rest, digestion, and repair. We'll dive deeper into the PNS in a few pages, but first, let's talk about the longer version of the sympathetic stress response.

The Stress Response: The Long Version

Imagine that you are now at the dinner table later that evening. You are half laughing about what happened earlier that day, when you thought, even if just for a few seconds, that your daughter was a burglar. You're feeling at ease when your phone lights up. You see a text message from your manager. Your company is currently undergoing a reorganization, and you know that half of you will be let go. In the last six months, the atmosphere has changed into a tense one, and you find yourself worrying throughout the day and ruminating over whether you'll have a job six months from now. Over the last few months, you haven't slept well; you've been feeling tired in the morning but totally amped at night. You've stopped exercising because of the tiredness, and that's led to some back pain and frequent headaches. Looking at the text, you feel that familiar prickle of stress, and your mind starts racing. Although lower in intensity, it feels a lot like the one you felt earlier today, when you heard the footsteps.

Once the adrenaline of the short-term acute stress response subsides, there begins a second wave of activity in the brain and body, which stimulates the release of the main stress hormone, cortisol. Cortisol's main job is to help the body deal with prolonged stress, and it keeps the sympathetic nervous system switched "on" by regulating energy metabolism, inflammation, the immune system, blood sugar levels, and digestion.

It may seem like the stress of a potential burglar in your home would be more damaging to your physiology than a simple text from your boss, but actually, ongoing low-grade stress is the most dangerous kind. The body doesn't distinguish between an actual physical

STRESS AND SICKNESS: Have you ever been sick at the beginning of your holiday? You aren't alone. This is incredibly common, and often occurs because the body—rushing to get prepared for your holiday and finish all your personal and professional to-dos—is in a state of chronic sympathetic activation. In this state, the body constantly releases cortisol, keeping you going through what your body interprets as an "emergency." But the moment you finally relax, the cortisol subsides, leaving you to deal with all the leftover effects of stress and chronic inflammation, and the sickness kicks in.

danger or the perceived "danger" of the mind. The mind has been hijacked, causing a mind-body disconnect. When we experience this stress chronically, the body will "adapt" to these less-than-ideal conditions by producing cortisol, oxidative stress, and inflammation, which are linked to just about every chronic health condition that exists. This has deadly consequences for human health worldwide, since emotional stress is a main contributing factor to the six leading causes of death, and studies show that 75 to 90 percent of doctor visits are for stress-related issues. Stress affects all systems of the body, including the musculoskeletal, respiratory, cardiovascular, endocrine, gastrointestinal, nervous, and reproductive systems, and is linked to:

- Anxiety
- Depression
- Digestive problems
- Headaches
- Thyroid issues
- Muscle tension and pain
- Heart disease, heart attack, high blood pressure, and stroke

- Sleep problems
- Weight gain
- Problems with memory and focus
- Hormonal imbalance, menstruation issues, and infertility
- Chronic inflammation and autoimmune disease
- Allergic disease such as allergies, eczema, and asthma
- Low libido
- Increased risk of infections

The WHM's ability to reduce stress may explain its benefit for so many diseases.

THE STRESS–WEIGHT GAIN CONNECTION: Nearly every woman had a moment in their life when they came home from a long, stressful day and instead of taking the time to cook a meal, we grabbed snacks and nervously started to eat our way out of a bag of chips or a bucket of ice cream. Stress eating, which is more prevalent among women, can cause us to gain weight. Sleep deprivation can also give you sugar and carb cravings because of a lack of energy. Further aggravating the weight gain is that you need to be out of an activated SNS and in "rest and digest" to trigger your metabolism.

We want to be clear: all this stress is not women's fault, despite women often being painted negatively as "worriers" or "uptight." Women's brains are biologically designed to pay more attention to potential threats than men's. Anticipating danger was how we would survive back in the caveman days! But these days, we have too many low-grade worries, and our brains are constantly ready to fight, flee, or freeze.

WOMEN AND STRESS: FROM NURTURE TO NATURE

If there were a competition for highest stress levels between the sexes, women would be the clear-cut winners. Women *are twice as likely* to suffer from severe stress, anxiety, and depression as men. According to the American Psychological Association, this "stress gap" gets bigger every year, with women consistently reporting higher and higher stress levels compared to men.

The explanation for this is a combination of genetics, physiology, environment, societal expectations, gender stereotypes, and learning. What a mix! Let's dive into some of these factors, starting with one of the most important: a lack of understanding and investment in women's health research.

- LACK OF RESEARCH: Excluding women from medical research has also hurt our knowledge of the female nervous system. While research shows women and men tend to react in a similar way to acute stressors, such as avoiding being hit by a car or hearing those footsteps upstairs, the female nervous system responds differently to chronic stressors. In recent years, it has been theorized that women have an additional stress response, called the "tend and befriend" response. This theory was introduced in 2000 by Shelley Taylor—a researcher at the Department of Psychology at UCLA—while the fight-or-flight response was first named in 1915 by Walter Cannon. It took eighty-five years to update our knowledge of the nervous system to be more applicable to ladies, and it's likely the first time you're hearing about it since this theory is only just beginning to be recognized. This theory is based on women's tendency to "keep the peace" by internalizing problems. While men seem to externalize stress (explode), women tend to internalize stress (implode). This may be due to differences in the structure and behavior of the brain.

- A MORE STRESS-SENSITIVE BRAIN: The brain is responsible for interpreting when there's a threat, and one thing that has become clear is that women's brains are more plastic, meaning they are more malleable and able to change. They are also smaller by about 150 grams and have more neural connections. The neurons are also much more active in female brains, with more parts lighting up during problem-solving, suggesting a higher level of connectivity and a more holistic use of the brain. The female prefrontal cortex, which is the most analytical and conscious part of the brain, also has a stronger connection to the amygdala, which is known as the fear center. Women also have more activity in the limbic regions, which include the amygdala, during stressful episodes. There are many upsides to these brain differences, but the downside of all this interconnectedness and activity is that the effects of external situations leave a larger imprint on female brains. Acute stress can become chronic stress much more easily.

- SILENT LABOR: Our work-life balance as women has changed drastically in just a few decades. Women have increasingly become part of the workforce but are often still expected to manage the majority of household tasks, such as child-rearing, cleaning, shopping, and cooking. This is often referred to as "silent labor" and adds to the physical and mental burden on women, leading to burnout, exhaustion, feelings of inadequacy, and overwhelm. Studies show that on average, women have five fewer hours of leisure time per week than men.

- SOCIAL/CULTURAL EXPECTATIONS: Not only are women busier than ever, balancing both work and home, but traditionally, they are expected to not complain about their load and therefore often deal with it by pretending that everything is fine. Women are expected to be sweet, kind, caring, and ladylike. To be of service. It is a socialized gender role for women to be highly agreeable, and this leads them to mask their feelings as they're expected to do more "nonpromotable work"—such as training new hires, planning team celebrations, or taking notes in meetings—and to not reveal their inner turmoil. Most women can relate to the feeling of talking to their boss and not being able to express their grievances, or finding it difficult to speak up during a meeting or to negotiate their salary. Both at home and at work, women seem to pay the price of doing more unacknowledged work for less recognition and less financial compensation.

- WORKPLACE INEQUALITY: On average, women working full-time, year-round, are paid 84 percent of what men are paid in equal positions. Studies show that women spend more time than men on nonpromotable tasks that are integral to the workplace, but that won't lead to a promotion due to lack of visibility and clear impact to the company's bottom line. This silent labor is expected, but does not come with recognition or financial compensation.

- BURNOUT: In our workshops, we see a lot more women than men recovering from burnout and suffering from low energy. Women have a heightened risk of burnout, and the COVID-19 pandemic has only increased this risk further. Since 2019, the number of women suffering from burnout has more than doubled.

- LESS SLEEP: Women are busier than ever, and while they actually need more sleep than men, they tend to get much less of it. Women get less deep rest, experience lower-quality sleep, and are 40 percent more likely to experience insomnia.

- VIOLENCE AGAINST WOMEN AND TRAUMA: There's no arguing with the fact that women must be constantly vigilant about their safety. Globally, an estimated 736 million women— almost one in three—have been subjected to physical and/or sexual intimate partner violence, nonpartner sexual violence, or both at least once in their life, and this figure does not include sexual harassment. Traumatic events have a tremendous amount of influence on our nervous system and stress response. Each one of us has an individual stress response, which is based on past experiences. When you carry a trauma, it makes you more stress-sensitive, and the body will react more quickly and more intensely to a stressful event, since the body is in a constant state of vigilance. This response can even span generations, as it makes an imprint on your genes, and especially travels through generations in marginalized communities, with women in these communities carrying the biggest burden.

- FEMALE HORMONES: Until puberty, men and women have the same stress response. Afterward, it seems the increase in sex hormones might play a role in the divergent responses to stress between men and women. Research by leading neurobiologist Bruce McEwen at the Rockefeller University showed that chronic stress caused shrinkage of certain parts of the brain and a loss of neurons in male animals; female animals, however, did not show the same shrinkage and actually had an increase in neural connections within the amygdala. But here's the interesting part: This only happened in the presence of estrogen. Without estrogen, the effects were the same in the male and female animals. Other research confirms this, showing that female rats have a more robust neuroendocrine response due to circulating estrogen levels, which increase stress hormone levels during and after both life-threatening and non-life-threatening stressors.

Women are faced with a dangerous combination of biological and societal factors that create a storm of chronic stress. Luckily, we have a built-in stress-fighting mechanism that's expertly designed to help us recover from and combat chronic stress.

WHM AND THE DE-STRESS BUTTON

No organism is designed to endure prolonged periods in a high-stress state. Rest and relaxation are nonnegotiable for a healthy body and mind, and recovery from stress is crucial. This is where the parasympathetic nervous system (PNS) comes into play. Originating in the brain stem, the parasympathetic nervous system acts like a car's brake pedal, providing a counterbalance to the effects of the SNS. The PNS works to stimulate the digestive and immune systems, reduce pupil size and heart rate, and contract the lungs. In a parasympathetic state, inflammation, stress hormones, and oxidative stress are cleared and the brain can rest, process information, and build new connections. In times of rest, the parts of the brain that modulate emotional regulation, creativity, and imagination finally light up.

One of the most important aspects of the parasympathetic nervous system is the vagus nerve. Known as the "wandering" nerve, the vagus nerve is the longest nerve in the body and runs from the base of the skull through the essential organs, including the lungs, heart, diaphragm, stomach, neck, throat, eyes, and ears. It plays a crucial role in regulating involuntary bodily functions, such as heart rate, digestion, respiratory rate, and immune responses. In our journey to get out of a sympathetic state and combat chronic stress, the vagus nerve is one of our most important tools. This is because certain practices, such as exercise, humming and singing, deep breathing, and (you guessed it!) cold exposure can stimulate the vagus nerve and jump-start the PNS. Currently, scientists are even working on creating devices that can stimulate the vagus nerve, but you can activate it naturally.

We already possess the tools we need to combat chronic stress. The WHM simply helps us activate these mechanisms that are already brilliantly built into our physiology, leading to an extremely effective antidote to chronic stress.

ENERGETIC CALMNESS: When Wim Hof broke the world record for sitting in ice in 2007, he gained insights into the vagus nerve. The author of the study, Dr. Tracey, suggested that Wim had likely learned to influence his autonomic nervous system, specifically by consciously engaging his vagus nerve. During the world record attempt, blood samples were taken before and after Wim spent two hours in the ice. Remarkably, the blood results revealed alterations consistent with deep vagus nerve stimulation, indicating a marked increase in parasympathetic activity, alongside a significant release of adrenaline, which is typically associated with sympathetic activation.

This dual response is a fascinating outcome of practicing the Wim Hof Method. On the one hand, you experience deep calm and restfulness, while on the other, you feel sharp and energized—we like to call it an "energetic calmness." This dynamic balance also explains the method's effectiveness in dealing with trauma. By inducing a controlled stressor, you can confront whatever emotions while remaining calm through vagus nerve activation. This creates a unique opportunity to reshape your relationship with fear and stress.

RESEARCH ON THE WHM AND STRESS

Even from the very first study on the WHM, it wasn't difficult to see immediately improvements in stress levels. The participants—the eighteen brave men who agreed to go to the highest mountains of Poland with Wim for the Radboud study—were dancing joyfully to the Harlem Shake, half-naked despite the freezing temperatures. Since that very first study, there's been quite a bit more investigation into the benefits of the WHM for stress.

One study showed that the WHM lowered stress in members

of an Antarctic expedition, which, due to long periods of isolation and extreme conditions, is known to cause considerable psychological stress. The participants started practicing the WHM one month before the expedition and continued it for a total duration of eight weeks, including some of the time they were on the expedition. They showed reduced psychological stress levels and an increase in the sleep hormone melatonin, which can be impaired by stress, compared to those who did not practice the WHM. The authors concluded that the Wim Hof Method "may positively affect stress symptoms and adaptability of the hormonal system to respond adequately to the circadian rhythm." In another study, published in *Brain Behavior and Immunity Integrative* in 2024, practicing the WHM for just six weeks positively impacted brain markers associated with stress resilience and regulation.

Several more studies have tested the effects of the WHM on stress in women. In one, sixty-one out of the ninety-nine subjects studied were female, and the results showed that practicing the WHM for two weeks lowered stress levels significantly. The results were most pronounced for the group that practiced the breathing, cold exposure, and mindset practices together, attesting to the synergistic effect of the three pillars to combat stress. In a retrospective survey by RMIT University completed on more than 3,000 WHM practitioners from different countries and backgrounds (411 of whom were women), roughly one-third reported significant benefits to their stress levels. Another study was done in conjunction with the psychiatric department at UCSF. The results also showed that three weeks of practicing the WHM lowered stress levels. This study was done only on female participants, and the results showed that the participants experienced long-term mental health benefits even when they discontinued their WHM practice, and even showed superior results to HIIT workouts in producing positive emotions.

At this point you might be wondering: How can sitting in an

ice bath possibly lead to *less stress*? Sitting in freezing water sounds incredibly stressful! It may seem like a direct contradiction, but it actually does lead to less stress due to a phenomenon called hormetic stress, or "positive" stress.

Hormetic Stress

Research tells us that a potent way to build stress resilience is by, somewhat ironically, introducing controlled, short-term stressors. After reading about the dangers of stress on the previous pages, this might come as a surprise. But hormetic stress is actually a well-studied and widely accepted concept in health and medicine. When confronted by an acute short-term stressor—one that in a higher dose or for a more prolonged period of time would be harmful—our bodies initiate an adaptive response. Over time, this actually leads to changes in cellular and molecular pathways that allow you to withstand stress more easily. The best example of hormetic stress is exercise. During exercise, the body experiences short-term thermal, metabolic, hypoxic, oxidative, and mechanical stress, but in response, it adapts, increasing overall muscular and cardiovascular capacity. The result? You become physically stronger and more resilient. Pretty soon, you're able to do with ease the exercise that once left you exhausted and sore. Other examples of hormetic stress include:

- Learning a new skill and/or completing a mental challenge
- Intermittent fasting
- Sauna
- Bungee jumping
- Public speaking

You can see what all these things have in common; they may be challenging in the moment and require some resilience and concentration, but they're incredibly rewarding in the long term, making you a stronger, healthier, more well-rounded person.

Studies show that hormetic stress can lead to the following physical and mental benefits:

- Upregulating adaptive stress response
- Strengthening resilience on a cellular level
- Improving physical condition and cognitive function
- Activating tissue and cellular renewal
- Regulating hormone production and levels
- Supporting the immune system
- Increasing energy

Engaging in these practices is the perfect antidote to our ultra-comfortable modern lifestyles. Because while we are more stressed than ever in some ways—with long workdays, sedentary lifestyle, economic and financial stress, low-nutrient diet, and hours of social media, TV, and the news cycle—we are also more comfortable than at any time in history. Many of us don't have to walk thousands of steps for water or food. We don't have to withstand hunger, cold, heat, or physical exhaustion. We almost always have a jacket, a snack, or a place to sit. If we don't want to do something difficult, challenging, or outside our comfort zone, there's a good chance we can find a way around it. One of the main underlying principles of the WHM is hormetic stress—the method challenges our bodies to make ourselves stronger for the next time.

With the WHM, we consciously use stress to de-stress. We practice increasing the space between the stressor and our response, making us more able to respond instead of react. You'll often hear us say "relax into the stress" or "bless the stress" to our students during the ice bath portion of our trainings and workshops, which is key to stress resilience.

As explained in the book *The Stress Prescription*, "acceptance" toward one's feelings and thoughts, especially negative experiences that we typically push away, is the key to increasing our stress resilience. People who practice awareness of their thoughts and feelings but also acceptance over their emotional and mental state experience improvements in stress reactivity, indicating that "acceptance" leads to greater stress resilience. When we not only endure the cold but also embrace and accept the feelings accompanying it, we increase our stress resilience. As our dad likes to say: "When stress comes knocking at your door, invite it in, embrace it, and then kick 'em out the door."

When you learn to consciously take control of stress with confidence, it's accompanied by downstream physical benefits that promote a state of health and balance throughout the body, as chronic stress is a contributing factor in almost all illnesses and diseases. This is particularly important for women, who experience hormone fluctuations that make them more sensitive to stress and its health consequences.

3

GO WITH THE FLOW: THE ENDOCRINE SYSTEM AND HORMONAL BALANCE

"Like the ocean moves in tune with the moon, women move with the current of our cycle."

We simply can't talk about the Wim Hof Method, women's health, or stress without discussing the important role hormones play in all three. The endocrine system, the system responsible for creating and releasing hormones in the body, is deeply connected to our nervous system. In fact, when we talk about the nervous system, we might as well refer to it as the neuro-endocrine system. Although separated in the past, looking at them symptomatically, these systems are inter-related and have to be approached holistically. When we affect one of those systems, it impacts all. When you influence the nervous system, you also influence the hormonal system, and all other systems connected to it.

So, before we dive deeper into the three pillars of the Wim Hof

Method—cold, breath, and mindset—it's important for us to understand the hormone system and the main female hormones. Let's dive into this magical, mysterious system occurring within us.

BREAKING DOWN THE ENDOCRINE SYSTEM

The endocrine system and nervous system have some similarities—for one, they both regulate the connection between body and mind—but they also have important differences. While the nervous system sends electrical signals via neurons, the endocrine system secretes hormones via glands that act as chemical messengers. While electrical messages via the nervous system go fast like electricity, and are more localized and short-term, the hormones we release move slower, spread through the body in the blood, and tend to linger much longer. They serve as powerful chemical messengers that intertwine to coordinate different functions throughout the body.

When most people think about hormones, puberty, the menstrual cycle, or pregnancy probably come to mind. But hormones are about so much more than reproduction. The endocrine system secretes hormones that act all over the body—in the organs, skin, muscles, and other tissues. Hormones don't just cause acne during puberty or nausea during pregnancy, they influence our thinking, our emotions, our physical well-being, and our behavior. In fact, humans have about fifty different hormones that are constantly being secreted, like an orchestra inside our body, regulating functions such as:

- Metabolism
- Growth and development
- Blood pressure
- Blood sugar levels
- The stress response

- Electrolyte and fluid balance
- Body temperature
- Sexual function
- Reproduction
- The sleep-wake cycle
- Mood

For example, the hormones cortisol and adrenaline regulate our stress response, while melatonin regulates our sleep cycle; hormones such as leptin and ghrelin control hunger and satiety signals; and insulin and glucagon regulate blood sugar levels. There is even a group of hormones called the "feel-good" hormones—including serotonin, dopamine, oxytocin, and endorphins—that regulate pleasure, motivation, and happiness. When our hormones are in balance, it contributes to our general health, so we feel good in our body and mind. But when the level of even one hormone becomes too high or too low, it can work against our health and cause an array of negative side effects.

Hormones are secreted by glands located all over the body that act as control centers, helping the nervous system and hormone system communicate to maintain homeostasis. To do this, they either upregulate or downregulate certain bodily functions depending on what's needed. Most hormones in the body are controlled by a negative feedback loop, which means that when a hormone is released, it sends feedback back to the gland to decrease its production. This helps make sure hormone levels never get too high or too low. When the delicate balance of hormones is disrupted, it can cause issues all over the body. You've probably heard of common female hormone issues, such as polycystic ovary syndrome (PCOS) and premenstrual dysphoric disorder (PMDD), but other common diseases affecting men and women—such as hyper- or hypothyroidism, diabetes, and obesity—are also caused by hormone imbalances.

MEET THE "FEEL-GOOD" HORMONES

1. Serotonin is produced when we feel content or satisfied. It can also be triggered by simple pleasures, like appreciating a beautiful sunset and realizing that happiness can be found in small moments. Serotonin levels tend to drop in winter due to a lack of vitamin D, which is needed to activate tryptophan, a precursor to serotonin. This is why some people experience the "winter blues," and in more severe cases, seasonal affective disorder (SAD). This is why I (Laura) take an extra winter dip when it gets really dark; it helps me whistle my winter blues goodbye! It is remarkable to think that 80 percent of your serotonin is made in the gut, and that our vagus nerve, which we can stimulate through deep breathing, extends from our brain to our gut.

2. Oxytocin, often called the "love hormone" or "love drug," is released during bonding activities, like breastfeeding or when you cuddle up on the couch with a loved one. It fosters feelings of love, warmth, and safety. As Harvard professor and hormonal expert Dr. Sara Gottfried outlines in her book *The Hormone Cure*, oxytocin acts as the anti-stress hormone that women desperately need to buffer against stress and counteract the effects of cortisol. It is produced when we feel safe, love, trust, empathy, forgiveness, but also when we kiss, cuddle, and feel socially bonded. Oxytocin has been shown to directly lower inflammatory markers, such as IL-6 and TNF-α, which the WHM also lowers.

3. Dopamine is another key chemical, associated with motivation and reward. It's released when we anticipate something pleasurable, like a tasty meal or potential sexual activity. Dopamine drives motivation, learning, and excitement. In fact, studies show that mice lacking dopamine stop eating and give up on life. It's also responsible for addictive behaviors, as it en-

courages us to repeat actions that make us feel good, like pulling a slot machine lever, smoking, or indulging in sugary snacks.
4. Endorphins, known as the body's natural painkillers, have an analgesic effect and are released in response to stress or pain. They improve mood, reduce stress, and enhance feelings of well-being.

Hormone imbalances and conditions are more common in women. In part this can be attributed to the fact that unlike men's hormones, which only fluctuate minimally throughout the day, woman's hormones fluctuate pretty drastically each month and even more throughout different phases of our lives, leaving more room for things to go awry.

WOMEN AND HORMONES

In addition to the hormones involved in nonreproductive bodily functions, there are sex hormones that regulate our reproductive system. Throughout our lives as women, these hormones send us extremely valuable signals and influence our bodily functions, emotions, thinking, and behavior. They include:

- ESTROGEN: Estrogen is a collective name for a group of hormones, including estrone (the primary form of estrogen after menopause), estriol (the primary form of estrogen during pregnancy), and estradiol (the primary and most potent form of estrogen produced during reproductive years). Estrogens play a crucial role in puberty, the menstrual cycle, pregnancy, and other bodily functions, like regulating cholesterol levels, blood sugar levels, bone and muscle mass, skin elasticity, and brain function.

Estrogen levels increase significantly during puberty, which leads to typical female features like breasts and curves and keeps the vaginal walls thick, elastic, and lubricated. The decline in estrogen during menopause is what causes symptoms like painful sex and vaginal dryness, and is also to blame for the large spike in health issues—like osteoporosis and heart disease.

If estrogen levels are too high, it can contribute to symptoms like irregular periods, menstrual bleeding, and dense breast tissue. High estrogen levels are also linked to a range of diseases, including breast and ovarian cancer, insulin resistance, and PCOS.

Estrogen has a strong effect on our mood. It's the equivalent of men's testosterone, the hormone that gets us ready for action. Estrogen also has an effect on serotonin production, which is one of the feel-good hormones.

- TESTOSTERONE: Testosterone may be the primary sex hormone in men, but women have plenty of it. In women, this hormone supports cognition, sex drive, and bone health. Low testosterone levels can cause weak bones, low libido, and fatigue. High testosterone levels can cause symptoms such as acne, male-pattern hair growth, irregular periods, and thinning hair.

- PROGESTERONE: Progesterone plays many important roles in women's health, including supporting mood, thyroid function, sleep, and inflammation. Progesterone levels fluctuate throughout your menstrual cycle, and its main role is to prepare the uterine lining so that a fertilized egg can implant and grow properly. If conception occurs, progesterone increases to support the pregnancy; if there's no fertilized egg, progesterone levels decrease and the uterine lining thins and breaks down, causing your period to start. It's uncommon to have too much progesterone, but low levels can cause symptoms such as irregular periods, breast tenderness, depression or mood changes, gallbladder issues, and low libido. If progesterone levels are low during pregnancy, it can contribute to miscarriage, preterm labor, and ectopic pregnancy.

Progesterone has a more calming effect on mood: your energy decreases and you may feel more introverted. As progesterone increases, you may also feel more relaxed and sleep better because it can stimulate calming neurotransmitters in the brain.

Together, estrogen and progesterone work like a duet to regulate the menstrual cycle.

The Menstrual Cycle

In addition to the circadian clock we discussed in the previous chapter, women have a second bodily clock: the menstrual cycle. The menstrual cycle is an infradian rhythm, a term that describes a bodily cycle longer than a single day. The menstrual cycle spans roughly twenty-eight days but can range anywhere from twenty-one days to thirty-five days. The menstrual cycle is separated into two phases— the follicular phase and the luteal phase—and is marked by fluctuations in sex hormones that cause changes to our body, all with the goal of bringing healthy offspring into the world.

The first part of the menstrual cycle, the follicular phase, consists of the first fourteen days of the cycle, starting with the first day of menstruation and ending at ovulation. All female hormones are at their lowest during menstruation, but then estrogen starts to rise steeply, signaling the lining of the uterus to grow. With the rise of estrogen, you also get an energy boost, improved mood, and feelings of increased well-being and confidence. Your desire to be outgoing and social is increasing thanks to the estrogen effect. Then, with the drastic rise in estrogen, an egg bursts out of its follicle, a small, fluid-filled sac inside the ovary where the egg grows and matures, and this marks ovulation. The length of the follicular phase depends on how long it takes the dominant follicle to form a fully matured egg and may vary at different stages of your life, ranging anywhere between ten and sixteen days.

With ovulation, the luteal phase begins. During ovulation, the body is biologically primed to be at its most vibrant and energetic, so you feel great during this (short) period. Then the released egg turns into something called the corpus luteum, which is a temporary gland that releases large amounts of progesterone and smaller amounts of estrogen. With the steady increase of progesterone, one will feel more calm and introverted. Under the influence of the progesterone, the lining of the uterus thickens for the possible fertilization of the egg. If the egg is not fertilized, levels of both estrogen and progesterone fall and bleeding begins, marking the beginning of the next cycle. The luteal phase is typically twelve to fourteen days long.

With all these hormone fluctuations going on under the surface, it's no wonder that women feel changes in their energy levels, mental health, and physiology throughout the month. Hormones are essential in ensuring that our natural rhythms run smoothly. Like the waves of the ocean ebb and flow, female hormones also rise and fall in tightly coordinated peaks and valleys. The menstrual cycle, with its fluctuating hormones, is not only about fertility. It is a reflection of a woman's health. It not only communicates with the body and mind but also influences our mood and behavior. If the hormones are in balance, they contribute to general health and well-being.

Recent research also shows the female brain changes dramatically during the different phases of the menstrual cycle, and our mood, memory, and behavior can change significantly.

Hormone Imbalance

If your hormones are at healthy levels, these monthly changes to mood and behavior may be minimal. But if you've got an imbalance in any of these hormones, the fluctuations may feel a lot more drastic, and you may experience unwanted symptoms. Everything in nature is fragile while in transition, so it makes sense that even small stressors could disrupt the intricate fluctuations of hormones in women's bodies. Unfortunately, our modern world is full of these small but constant stressors; chronic stress, low-nutrient food, a sedentary lifestyle, environmental toxins, and not enough time to rest and restore can significantly disrupt the delicate equilibrium of female hormones.

When this happens, your body will send you signals that it's out of whack, such as:

- Hair loss
- No sexual desire
- Poor sleep quality
- Mood changes
- Brain fog and less focus
- Skin changes
- Fatigue and low energy
- Persistent weight gain
- Hot flashes and sweats
- Infertility
- Breast discharge

These symptoms aren't always easy to make sense of, and many women spend years without any answers or support. Because of the lack of research, physicians are often uninformed about female hormone health, which means that women are left alone to do their own research. Western medicine—which tends to take a generalized, one-size-fits-all approach to health—just doesn't lead to effective treatments for women suffering from hormonal imbalances.

Hormone imbalance can also induce changes to the menstrual cycle. Because this cycle involves a complex interplay between the organs and hormones, it can act as a reflection of a person's overall health and hint if there's a problem. In fact, it's often referred to as the "fifth vital sign" that doctors should consider along with blood pressure, body temperature, heart rate, and respiratory rate. It's important to pay attention to any changes to the cycle, including:

- PREMENSTRUAL SYNDROME (PMS): Research shows that close to 80 percent of women have PMS issues and 50 percent seek medical help for them. Symptoms of PMS include depression, irritability, water retention, breast tenderness, headaches, abdominal pains, and mood swings.
- IRREGULAR CYCLES: This can mean irregularity in the amount of blood you lose, the number of days that you bleed, and/or the number of days between periods. Young women in puberty, women right after pregnancy, and women in perimenopause are more likely to have irregular cycles, and an estimated 14–25 percent of women experience this symptom of hormone imbalance.
- AMENORRHEA: Primary amenorrhea refers to someone not having their first period by age fifteen. Exposure to a host of hormonal disruptors has been shown to lead to hormone metabolism disorders during puberty, and may "play a role in accelerating or delaying the onset of menarche." Secondary amenorrhea is diagnosed when you have a period missing for more than three months. When secondary amenorrhea is not related to pregnancy, breastfeeding, or menopause, it is likely due to metabolic, physical, or psychological stress.
- PERIOD PAIN: Most women will experience period pains, also known as dysmenorrhea, in their lives. In fact, one survey showed that 85 percent of forty-two thousand girls in the US have painful cramps during their period. Another study found that for 20 percent of the women the pain is so severe that they cannot do regular activities.

We hear words like "cramps" and "PMS" all the time, but that doesn't make them less serious or debilitating. Hormone changes can lead to significant increases in anxiety and depression and even exacerbate psychiatric disorders. This research shows that during the luteal phase, anxiety, stress, and binge eating appear to be relatively more elevated. Strong evidence shows increases in psychosis, mania, depression, suicide/suicide attempts, and alcohol use during the premenstrual and menstrual phases.

These symptoms can also be linked to hormone-related illnesses, such as:

- endometriosis
- uterine fibroids
- polycystic ovary syndrome
- premature ovarian failure
- menstrual irregularity
- menarche
- infertility
- hyperthyroidism

Hormonal Shifts: Overcoming the Delicate Transitions

In addition to our regular monthly cycle, women also experience multiple major hormonal shifts during their lives: puberty, pregnancy, perimenopause, and menopause. These big transitions not only affect the reproductive system, but as neuroscientist Lisa Mosconi notes, we can better describe them as neuro-endocrine transitions, as the brain changes dramatically as well. These transitions are marked by an increase in stress and inflammation, which can be balanced naturally if the adrenals are healthy and women are stress resilient and have a daily dose of anti-stress. Added to this is the fact that estrogen and progesterone, which have protective properties, decline in our thirties and forties, which then greatly magnifies the impact of stress and unhealthy lifestyles. These delicate hormonal transitions can also coincide with other major life events that act as chronic stressors, often the case with women in their thirties and forties. During this period, women are often faced with stressful life circumstances like unresolved trauma coming up to the surface, a high-pressure career, being a primary caretaker, losing a loved one, getting fired, or filing for divorce. Hormonal shifts are already destabilizing moments for our bodies; when we have additional stressors on top of it all, hormonal fluctuations are aggravated and there is limited opportunity for our hormones to rebalance. With the WHM, we take back control of the steering wheel by supporting the body's innate capacity to rebalance itself.

HORMONE DISRUPTORS

Our neuroendocrine systems have not had the time to adapt to the challenges of the modern world and the constant levels of stress, strain, and disruption. And when the body believes it is in a constant state of danger, it will produce continuous levels of cortisol and adrenaline. And while adrenaline and cortisol are amazing at dealing with challenges in the short term, in the long run, pumping out these hormones is not sustainable and can wreak havoc on female health.

If you've ever missed a period when you were stressed or sick, you've already experienced this connection for yourself. Too much stress will greatly affect a woman's menstrual cycle, as the body thinks it's in fight-or-flight mode and prioritizes survival over reproductive functions. Instead of sex hormones, the body will produce continuous levels of cortisol, which takes center stage and pushes all the other competing female hormones to the wings. Needing to produce so much cortisol creates a constant strain on our bodies and our health.

The Hierarchy of Hormones

To understand hormonal balance, it is imperative to know that there is a hierarchy in the production and balance of hormones. Just like in Maslow's hierarchy of needs, survival gets priority over everything. Survival is the basic need of every organism, so our bodies will always favor the hormones involved in the fight-flight-freeze responses. Below the hormones responsible for survival fall the hormones in charge of maintenance, such as thyroid and insulin. These regulate many important functions essential for optimal health, such as metabolism and digestion. Below that, we have functions involved in things like socializing, thriving, and reproducing, which involves hormones like estrogen, progesterone, and serotonin. This hierarchy of hormones makes it extremely simple to understand why hormone balances can be disrupted when we are stressed. Stress creates a constant strain on our bodies as it causes our bodies to inhibit other important functions in favor of survival.

Stress

As the stress system mediates the reproductive system, stress can impact the release of female hormones. This can have a big impact on female health, as it can lead to imbalances in hormones such as thyroid hormones, progesterone, estrogen, and testosterone and the delicate balance between them. Cortisol and female hormones have an intricate interplay that is easily upset. For example, when cortisol rises, estrogen will decline; when cortisol decreases, estrogen will increase. Another clear example of how cortisol can directly influence sex hormones involves progesterone. Progesterone and cortisol use the same nutritional building blocks. Because surviving is our body's priority, producing cortisol always comes first, which leaves less nutrition to build progesterone. This can affect the production of progesterone in the adrenals and even block some of the progesterone receptors. Too much cortisol can also lower the production of testosterone, a hormone that's often the culprit behind low libido. Research shows that psychological stress can affect the natural decrease and increase of estrogen during our cycle, making the ups and downs either more extreme or the opposite, more blunted. As one study notes, "Stress at any age leads to the depletion of estrogen and testosterone stores in the body."

Research shows that chronic stress in women can lead to menstrual irregularities, anovulation, absence of menstruation, and even infertility. One study showed that women with high stress levels were two to three times more likely to be infertile. For women in the higher stress group who did become pregnant, it took them more cycles to become pregnant. When our bodies feel unsafe, they decide it is not a time to procreate but to hide, withdraw socially, and be on alert for danger. Cortisol also interferes with the output and regulation of thyroid hormone, which has been linked to lower fertility or infertility. Millions of women in the US are affected by the overproduction or underproduction of thyroid hormone, which leads to many of the symptoms associated with female hormonal imbalance, such as fatigue, hair loss, anxiety, weight gain or loss, or even conditions that mostly affect women, such as fibromyalgia or Hashimoto's disease.

Stress also leads directly to chronic inflammation. When experiencing chronic stress, we release inflammatory proteins to detect a potential threat. As the authors of one study noted: "Almost any stage of inflammatory and immunological responses is affected by hormone actions." They crosstalk and affect one another, leading to changes in mood, behavior, and health. Chronic stress causes chronic inflammation and can even shut down systems designed to heal, restore, and reproduce. One study reported that women with high levels of inflammation had a 24 to 41 percent increase in most PMS symptoms. Research from 2022 seems to confirm this connection, linking higher levels of inflammation to PMS and PMDD. Even period pain is related to inflammation. Cramps are caused by an increase in levels of prostaglandins, which play a hormone-like role in regulating bodily processes and are part of the inflammatory response to injuries. Research has established a link between stress, cramps, and prostaglandin concentrations.

As we'll learn in Chapter 8, inflammation is at the root of most major diseases affecting modern humans, so it's important to know how to break this cycle of stress, inflammation, and hormone imbalance. The interplay between stress, inflammation, and hormone imbalance is extremely complex, and a lot is simply unknown about the exact ways these factors combine to impact women's health negatively. More studies need to be done on female hormonal imbalance and its impact on our health and well-being. What we do know is that energy being diverted for survival is also the energy that could be spent on restoring and rebalancing our hormonal balance.

Insulin and Ghrelin

Prolonged cortisol production also increases the risk of insulin resistance, another major disruptor of female hormonal balance and health. Cortisol floods the body with glucose, which is sent to the muscles to provide them with quick energy to fuel the fight-or-flight response. While this is an amazing tool to prepare us for emergency situations, if it happens chronically, it can lead to insulin resistance as the body simply can't keep up with the metabolic demand. Insulin resistance often leads to weight gain, which creates a snowball effect among women suffering from hormonal imbalances, as being overweight also leads to excess estrogen and inflammation. While women are gaining weight, they have cells that are craving glucose but can't absorb it due to the insulin resistance. This results in women feeling extremely tired and reaching for high-calorie foods full of sugar, fat, and salt. As Dr. Elizabeth Blackburn and Dr. Elissa Epel note in their book *The Telomere Effect*: "Chronic stress can lead to overeating, co-elevation of cortisol and insulin, and suppression of certain anabolic hormones. This state of metabolic stress in turn promotes abdominal adiposity. Both the direct stress response and the accumulation of visceral fat can promote a milieu of systemic inflammation and oxidative stress."

Similarly, when women experience stress, the hunger hormone ghrelin is produced, and that increases hunger and thoughts about food—especially low-nutrient, highly addictive and tasty ones that we are at high risk of overeating. Put all this together and it leads to an increase in visceral fat, which in turn is associated with the release of low-grade inflammation. Fat storage also leads to the secretion of more cortisol, which creates a vicious cycle of cortisol and weight gain. A vast array of female hormonal conditions have been linked to insulin resistance, and because estrogen, which has a protective role against insulin resistance, decreases in perimenopause and menopause, women in these stages should be extra cautious about insulin resistance.

And it's not just stress that affects hormones, either. There are other hormone disruptors we should be aware of.

Environmental Hormone Disruptors

Psychological stress can clearly impact health, but environmental and lifestyle factors only add to the stress-inflammation–hormone imbalance cycle. In addition to psychological stress, we are bombarded with hormonal disruptors in our cleaning products, cosmetics, clothes, and menstrual products. We are exposed to pollution in the air, water, and food in the form of microplastics, heavy metals, and pesticides. We call these "hormone disruptors" because these chemicals are known to cause inflammation and mimic, block, or alter the natural production of certain hormones, leading to their over- or underproduction.

Common hormone disruptors include:

- Parabens: A group of chemicals that are used in the food and drinks industry, as well as in beauty and personal care products.
- Pesticides: Found in Roundup and other gardening products
- Bisphenol A: Found in plastic products, like Tupperware containers
- Phthalates: Found in common cosmetics
- Triclosan: Found in common types of soap
- Polychlorinated biphenyls: Found in industrial and consumer products

These hormonal imbalances can even travel across generations, impacting the fetus if the mother is exposed to them during pregnancy. We are most sensitive to these disruptors during hormonal shifts, such as puberty, our monthly cycle, pregnancy and postpregnancy, and through perimenopause and menopause.

Research clearly shows that certain foods can be hormone disruptors as well. Studies have connected sugar, dairy, refined grains, red meat, and processed foods to higher levels of estrogen in women, lower levels of testosterone in men, and even insulin and cortisol imbalance.

IS THE PILL A HORMONE DISRUPTOR? Similarly, hormonal contraceptives, such as the birth control pill, mimic certain female hormones, leading to disruptions and increased risk of some cancers, anxiety, and depression. A recent study of 131 women on the pill showed that the pill interfered with the body's ability to regulate stress, and negatively impacted the female stress response. What is clear is that these hormonal disruptors lead to hormonal imbalances, as they interfere with the normal functioning of our endocrine system. They may also block the body's natural production of hormones needed to maintain homeostasis.

THE WHM FOR HEALTHY HORMONES

You might be wondering: Are hormone imbalances and the symptoms and illnesses that accompany them just a burden women are destined to bear? The answer is no! Our bodies were designed for hormonal harmony, not hormonal chaos.

To support hormone balance, we recommend starting with the foundations, which will reduce your exposure to hormone disruptors and allow your body to shift out of the survival state and help it to prioritize reproduction and repairs.

- Minimizing the use of hormonal disruptors by eating organic and using nontoxic products
- Minimizing sugar in the diet
- Physical exercise
- Prioritizing sleep

These steps can help us reduce inflammation and detox from harmful substances and maintain an ecosystem that is as healthy as possible. In addition to these lifestyle tips, the Wim Hof Method works directly on the body to rebalance hormones and reduce inflammation.

The WHM can work to counteract the effects of hormone disruptors by engaging the arterial muscles, improving blood flow, and flushing the arteries and lymphatic system. The lymphatic system is key to the immune system—with over eight hundred small lymph "nodes" distributed throughout the body that work to transport white blood cells—and needed for detoxifying from excess hormones, toxins, and inflammation byproducts, and clearing waste from our bodies. Like the cardiovascular system, the lymphatic system transports fluid around the body using tiny vascular muscles. But instead of blood, the fluid is lymph; about five liters of this clear fluid is circulated throughout the body daily. Both deep breathing and cold exposure bolster the lymphatic system, supporting immune health and the body's detoxification mechanisms.

Hormonal transitions are already marked by lowered stress resilience, so more burden to the system during these times can be very impactful. The most important factor, then, is the WHM's ability to counteract psychological and physiological effects of stress because it deals with the root cause of hormone imbalance, as we switch the body from "survive" mode to "restore" mode. When we are in a more restful state, we allow our body to focus on more than just survival, and switch to focus on repairing and restoring itself, and rebalancing our hormones. If we can help our bodies maintain homeostasis, and increase stress resilience (through allostasis), we are helping them reestablish hormonal order. By changing our biochemistry through the breathing exercises and cold exposure, we give our nervous system a reset, and thus, we give our endocrine system a reset as well. In one study into the Wim Hof Method with a small sample size that included women, the reset of the hormonal system was underlined with regard to the stress hormone cortisol and melatonin. The authors concluded that the "WHM can improve the adaptability of the hormonal system." This study confirms changes to hormones related to the circadian rhythm, but it also points to the principle that the hormonal system can adjust and adapt with the help of the WHM. To de-stress is to clean up toxins, reduce inflammation, and balance hormones. We break the vicious cycle and return to our natural state of hormone harmony. We also optimize the body's ability to handle stress, and create a higher mental resilience toward stress, an essential part in dealing with the stress women encounter during their major life and hormonal transitions, when the impact of stress can hit them harder.

As WHM instructors who talk with thousands of women practicing the method, we've seen firsthand how many of them see improvements in hormone imbalances. They often report:

- A decrease in or elimination of pain during menstrual cycles
- A regular cycle instead of an unpredictable one
- Improvements in female conditions such as endometriosis and PCOS
- Better mood regulation during PMS
- Fewer emotional highs and lows
- Higher libido
- Improved energy levels
- Easier transitions into menopause, pregnancy, and postpartum

In later chapters, we'll dive into the benefits of the WHM for specific conditions related to inflammation, hormone imbalance, and the immune and lymphatic systems. But first, we'll talk about the method itself and exactly why the combination of cold, breath, and mindset is so powerful for improving women's health.

THE CHEMISTRY BETWEEN WOMEN AND ICE

"The best way to balance the strong, masculine force of the cold is with the soft, feminine approach of embracing it and letting go."

For as long as three thousand years, the legendary Ama, also known as the sea women of Japan, have been diving into cold waters, scouring the bottom of the ocean for seafood and pearls to bring home. This profession was considered a sacred undertaking and over the decades, the Ama became conditioned to the sometimes near-freezing temperatures. Diving into deep waters from the age of twelve to sometimes seventy or eighty years old, the Ama learned how to control their body temperature and stay warm against all odds. We love to think about the similarities between the Ama and the pearls they spent thousands of years collecting: Pearls are created when a mollusk launches a defense process against an irritant, like sand. For the Ama, the challenge of the cold activates that same defense process that helps them adapt, unleashing their inner strength. According to historical documents, women were considered the natural choice for this role because of their higher body fat content. And now we know that fat can actually act as an insulating layer, giving women an edge when facing the cold.

Today, in our WHM workshops and Icewomen meetings, we welcome ladies of all ages, backgrounds, and levels of experience with the cold. (With one of the oldest WHM practitioners being a wonderful ninety-five-year-old woman who was taught by her ninety-seven-year-old sister!) And what we have learned through years of witnessing women interact with the cold is that it gives them a deeper and more powerful connection with themselves, one where outside noise is immediately silenced. Despite often being hesitant about walking into a WHM training—not necessarily because of the ice bath itself but the idea of showing up, stripping down to a bikini in front of a group of strangers, and doing something completely out of their comfort zone—women are far more resilient than they think.

We have been blown away by the number of women who, the minute they realize they can overcome the fear of the cold, start to trust themselves and feel more empowered. After years of leading WHM trainings, the two biggest surprises in the ice bath section of our training are always: 1) the overly confident men and 2) the hesitant ladies. We have seen dozens of Arnold Schwarzenegger types go confidently toward the ice bath, only to have their egos crushed as they squeal and squirm trying to stay in. We have seen just as many ladies brimming with anxiety before they do their first ice bath, only to discover that they are far more resilient than they expected, often entering a state of Zen on the very first immersion. We see far more female anxiety before the ice bath, and far more male anxiety during the ice bath.

During many of Wim's events, after everyone has their first "official" ice dip led by Wim and the instructors, there are some people who stay in the ice bath a little longer or go in again. We call them the "after-partiers"—and they are mostly women! The women really seem to enjoy being together as a social gathering, which strengthens their ability to stay in the cold longer. The result is like a secret, girls-only (iced) tea party. Like the Ama, all women have a sacred bond with the cold that only needs to be accessed to come to life.

But what exactly explains this sacred connection between women and the cold? And what lessons can the cold teach women? We are asked these questions all the time. To form answers, we must consider both the real-life experiences of women and scientific facts, starting with the major system at play when we step into the cold—the cardiovascular system.

OUR BODIES AND THE COLD

Cardiovascular disease is the leading cause of death for women globally, and the reason for this is rooted in our modern lifestyles. With air-conditioning in the summer and heat in the winter, our daily routines fail to stimulate this system, which leads to weakening over time. But the cold enables us to reignite the potential of this incredible system that runs on the beating of our hearts. When we do cold exposure, we are actually training this invisible infrastructure of 125,000 kilometers of blood vessels, arteries, and a heart that pumps six liters of blood constantly throughout our bodies. If you dissected a human body and opened all the veins and arteries, placing them side to side, you could go around the world 2.5 times. That is how intricate this system is. Each blood vessel in your body contains tiny smooth muscles that close (vasoconstrict) and open (vasodilate) to pump the oxygen-rich blood to every organ, tissue, and cell, and then pump the carbon dioxide–rich blood back to the lungs. When we go into the cold, the blood vessels constrict. When we warm up after, the blood vessels dilate. It's like going to the gym for a high-intensity vascular workout.

When the smooth muscles of the vascular system work well, they help the heart more effortlessly transport blood throughout the body, so your heart's workload is reduced—an instant stress reliever. A healthy vascular system also enables the efficient removal of toxins and waste, as well as plaque buildup in the arteries, which is a major cause of heart disease. When the blood flows efficiently, it also boosts your nervous system, as these vascular muscles open and close due to the motor function of the nerves (electricity). Just like your big muscles get a good workout at the gym, your little muscles get a workout with cold exposure. When we go into the cold, the arterial muscles of our veins and arteries contract and close. When we warm up after, these muscles help the veins open up. By engaging with the cold, we can train and tone this vast infrastructure: a complete vascular workout.

Laura: In our house, it wasn't the weatherman that decided what we wore—we always just went by how we felt. If I was cold, I'd tell my dad, and he'd give me a sweater or jacket. I remember a couple of times when my teacher told my dad to get me a jacket because it was supposedly too cold outside. At fourteen, I was oblivious to the changing seasons. I'd been taking cold showers since I was eleven, and one year I wore a tank top in the middle of winter. I never felt a significant shift as the seasons changed; I simply went by feeling, naturally transitioning and gradually adapting. Once, a girl at school walked up to me in the yard and rudely asked why I was wearing a tank top without a jacket. I understand her concern now, but back then, I just raised an eyebrow, finding her question odd. To me, the answer was obvious: I didn't feel cold!

And yet, we are taught from a young age to fear the cold. Our parents wrapped us in warm scarves and hats, telling us to stay inside to avoid "catching a cold." (Although as you can imagine, our dad would say the opposite: "Take the coats off, or you will get sick!") Willfully exposing ourselves to this powerful force of nature might seem crazy, but our bodies are incredibly intelligent and perfectly able to adapt to and handle colder temperatures. Ancient populations were able to inhabit places like Siberia and Alaska before electricity. It's just that the mind can interfere with the natural intelligence of our built-in capabilities shaped through millions of years of evolution to handle fluctuations in temperature. Of course, this doesn't mean we should throw away all our jackets, but we can condition ourselves to not instantly put on five layers the minute we feel a cool breeze.

Contrary to the false wisdom about the cold being bad for us, our bodies are expertly built to adapt to cold through a variety of mechanisms that regulate internal temperature.

Temperature Regulation

Our bodies have an amazing ability to regulate our internal body temperature, which is maintained at a cozy average of 98.6 degrees, fluctuating slightly depending on time of day and the individual. Our bodies evolved this way because 98.6 degrees is similar to the warmest external environments humans frequently encounter. With more options to warm up than cool down, our bodies prefer our internal temperature to be warmer than our external environment. Temperatures higher than 98.6 degrees can affect our biology negatively, so keeping to this average is ideal to maintain a healthy temperature balance.

When the external temperature goes up or down, our cardiovascular system and nervous system work together like a built-in heater and air conditioner directed by a part of the brain called the hypothalamus, which acts as a sort of coordinating center, to keep your body in a stable state of homeostasis. When the body is exposed to heat, the hypothalamus triggers vasodilation, which allows the blood vessels to open up so warm blood is distributed to the extremities, and heat is released through the skin to cool us down. If our body temperature stays too high, our brain gets a signal that it is time to take additional measures and our sweat glands activate, making sure our body temperature drops to a manageable level. This is all strictly regulated. Think about it: if you experience even a 1-degree increase in internal body temperature, you have a fever.

This same system activates when we're exposed to the cold. Directed by our hypothalamus, our bodies first turn to vasoconstriction, which reduces blood flow and increases the insulating capacity of the skin by closing pores. Vasoconstriction happens first in the hands, feet, arms, and legs in an effort to reduce the flow of warm blood away from the core body, preserving heat for the head and vital organs, which are more important for survival than the extremities. The more well-known example of this is frostbite. If you were to be enveloped in a snowstorm in Antarctica without proper equipment, your extremities would turn black and essentially "die." This is your body's way of protecting the core body and sacrificing nonvital parts of the body. It doesn't look pretty, but by preserving your core temperature, your heat preservation mechanisms will help you survive.

The process of heat preservation kicks into gear starting at 95 degrees in water compared to 78.8 degrees in air because water strips away heat more quickly than air. Interestingly, thermoreceptors and pain receptors are closely linked. This is why stepping into the cold can feel excruciatingly painful; your body is signaling to your brain that there is "danger" to its internal homeostasis and you should avoid whatever is going on. Pain is nothing but a signal to move you into action, in this case telling you to move to a warmer environment. This vasoconstriction begins when the skin temperature reaches

95 degrees and ramps up to maximum capacity when the skin temperature reaches 87.8 degrees or less.

In addition to heat preservation, we also have heat-producing mechanisms, which protect us against the cold by ramping up internal physiological processes that naturally produce heat, also known as metabolic processes. If you go into an ice bath, your body will work to not only preserve heat but produce it through one of these processes. Heat production involves multiple metabolic pathways that generate heat from carbohydrates, fats, and proteins. The one we lean on for heat production depends on which is the most energy-efficient, and that is based on someone's unique constitution and training. One way our bodies do this is through the activation of brown fat.

Brown Fat Activation

Most of our body fat is composed of white fat, the type of fat you're likely already familiar with. Compared to white fat, which stores extra energy, brown fat is metabolically more active, burning energy to produce heat. Because it acts more like muscle than fat, we often refer to it as "active fat." It contains more iron-rich mitochondria, which are the energy factories of our cells and provide a shortcut to producing heat when we're exposed to temperatures 60.8 degrees or lower. This occurs because the body releases the hormone norepinephrine in response to cold, which signals the mitochondria in the brown fat to increase energy output, generating instant heat.

Brown fat is critical for humans when we're first born. It protects babies from getting too cold when they haven't yet developed muscles, and obviously cannot put clothes on for themselves! It serves as a great survival mechanism to protect our youngest and most vulnerable and is specifically distributed in the body to protect the heart and brain. For years, researchers thought brown fat wasn't present after infancy, but in 2009, Dutch researchers proved otherwise. In other research, PET/CT scans showed that adults have about fifty grams of brown fat, and new discoveries about its functions are still being made. More recent research has also shown that through cold training, we can slowly convert white fat into brown fat. The activation of brown fat helps explain many of cold exposure's benefits to metabolic health, including increased metabolism and improved blood sugar health.

Brown fat isn't the only relevant pathway involved when it comes to heat production. In fact, an increase in muscle activity seems to be an even better way for the body to produce heat.

To Shiver or Not to Shiver? That Is the Question!

For humans, the most energy-efficient way to generate heat is through skeletal muscle contraction in the form of shivering, which allows you to quickly metabolize glucose and fatty acids to generate heat. This happens with microscopic shivering—which is invisible to the eye and happens without you even realizing it—or visible shivering, which happens when the core body temperature is sufficiently compromised. Visible shivering is an involuntary process where the muscles in the torso and the limbs take over and tremble uncontrollably to generate heat as a protective mechanism. This type of shivering can feel uncomfortable, like you've lost control of your body.

Recently, some people have even touted it as a way to lose weight, which has led to a trend where people engage in cold exposure way too many times and for way too long with the goal of getting their bodies to shiver like hell, thinking this is the right way to do it. We can't argue with the fact that physically, you might burn more calories when you shiver like crazy—your body is using a lot of energy to survive! However, extreme shivering is not necessary to get any of the benefits of cold exposure. You will still experience a considerable increase in metabolism without this type of shivering, as it's also a sign of a mind-body disconnect as your body takes over, which is the opposite of the goal of the WHM. Uncontrollable shivering decreases with more training and a stronger mind-body connection. The conditioned response to cold training should be to feel in control over your physiology, connected with the body, and able to heat up gradually without uncontrollable shivering. We teach how to warm up by heating up from within and deepening the mind-body connection through breathing exercises, mindset practices, and physical poses and movements.

EXTREME COLD CONDITIONING: In 2008, at the hypothermia facility at the University of Minnesota, Wim's body temperature was observed during more than two hours of exposure to the cold. Normally, when exposed to extreme cold for long periods of time, humans suffer extreme vasoconstriction that automatically restricts blood flow to the extremities to protect the vital organs. The skin starts to tingle with a burning sensation or even a loss of sensation, and tissue death may set in. When the core body temperature falls below 95 degrees, hypothermia takes effect and the heartbeat, blood pressure, and respiration rate drop, causing the person to feel faint and weak, ultimately leading to loss of consciousness. After about an hour, unless there is an external source of heat to remedy the situation, the hypothermia will normally result in death.

But during the experiment in 2008, Wim's temperature dropped below 89.9 degrees for more than eighty minutes without these effects setting in. Incredibly, Wim increased his body temperature voluntarily—through breathing and mindset exercises he'd been honing for decades—from that 89.9 to 97.5 degrees all on his own, without an external source of heat. Dr. Ken Kamler, the lead hypothermia researcher and author of *Surviving the Extremes*, was baffled, saying: "It's a mystery that we have not yet come close to solving. It tells us that there's enormous potential within the brain that is going untapped. And if we can study him more, and study people like him more, maybe we can unleash that potential for the rest of us." Another study showed that during eighty minutes of cold water exposure, Wim's body temperature remained constant at 98.6 degrees, his heart rate remained low, and his blood pressure remained normal.

How is this physically possible? Multiple studies have examined Wim's superhuman response to the cold, including one in 2010 by Dr. Marianne Hopman from Radboud University. This study showed that Wim's metabolic rate increased by 300 percent as he sat in a bucket of ice, submerged to his neck. Dr. Hopman noted that Wim didn't shake or shiver, concluding: "We don't understand how this is possible." Another study by Maastricht University in 2014, showed that Wim produced 35 percent more body heat in a low-temperature environment of 51.8 degrees than at room temperature. This increase in his core body temperature even reached 50 percent during the experiment, compared to a 20 percent increase observed in other people in similar experiments.

Clearly, Wim can generate internal heat at rates far higher than the average person. At first, the head researcher, Dr. Wouter Lichtenbelt, thought maybe Wim had more brown fat than the average person, but when Wim was tested and compared to his twin brother, they found similar amounts of brown fat between them. It was a Michigan study in 2018 that finally brought to light the reason for Wim's incredible heat production. The researchers observed that the breathing exercises he did throughout the experiment caused his intercostal muscles, the muscles between the ribs, to absorb 300 percent more glucose, which was converted into heat. In this study, Wim was willfully controlling his body's heat production using his intercostal muscles and did not show any form of vasoconstriction, shivering, or hypothermia. In the same study, the researchers observed Wim's response to the cold with an fMRI scan. For this part of the experiment, he wasn't allowed to do any breathing exercises. Instead, Wim meditated and hummed, and surprisingly, his body warmed up like it had before. As Wim explains, "I visualized being in the same state when I was climbing Mount Everest or running a half marathon barefoot in shorts in freezing temperatures. I tapped into the potential of my physiology through my mind." The humming was a way for Wim to get into a meditative state even while he was surrounded by the distracting sounds of the machine. Humming also activates the vagus nerve and opens the veins, enabling warm blood to flow where the body needs it.

Wim is a highly trained individual, and it's important to keep in mind that these are extreme examples under scientific, controlled settings. That said, in these studies he was using the very same cold, breathing, and mindset exercises that we will teach you right here in this book!

When talking about how our bodies respond to the cold, we can't ignore some obvious gender differences. Women do experience the cold differently from men, and it could be one reason why they are more hesitant about the cold at first.

WOMEN AND TEMPERATURE:
COLD HANDS AND WARM HEARTS

For many women—after years of borrowing jackets, running home for a sweater, or powering through cold offices or freezing restaurants—it won't come as a surprise that research shows women have a clear preference for warmer environments. And it's not just a preference; there are actually biological differences that make women more sensitive to the cold.

The sensation of "feeling cold" is triggered by thermoreceptors in the skin and is actually based on the difference between the core body temperature and the temperature in the extremities. Research shows that women's hands are about 5.04 degrees colder and their core body temperature is 0.36 to 0.72 degrees higher on average compared to men, which means there is a bigger contrast between core body and hand and feet temperature at baseline, explaining why women feel colder. This explains the saying that women have "cold hands, warm hearts"! Women also have more robust vasoconstriction and greater nerve density at the skin level, which makes them more tuned in and sensitive to environmental stimuli, including temperature differences. TRPM8, a temperature-sensitive receptor in the skin that is activated around 77 degrees and acts as a stimulus for shivering, is more sensitive in women than men.

FEEL HOT, STAY WARM? One fascinating piece of research shows that self-perception can help determine how cold we feel. The study interviewed women waiting outside a nightclub on a cold evening and found that the more attractive they felt, the less physically cold they felt. How interesting is that! We can all channel Paris Hilton ("that's hot") whenever we want to boost our thermogenesis abilities.

This difference in temperature regulation has no doubt caused conflict over the years. Offices have their temperature set at around 71 degrees, a temperature that was determined as being "ideal" for the male body back in the 1960s. Women, however, are most comfortable and productive in temperatures 4.5 degrees warmer, according to a 2015 study by Dutch scientists, which clearly lines up with women's hands being 5.04 degrees colder than men's. Since the 1960s, women have increasingly joined the workplace, but only 35 percent of office buildings have adjusted their temperatures. The researchers of one study said that this "overcooling" of offices points to a clear gender inequality. The body is always working to preserve energy, so if it is working hard to maintain a warm enough internal temperature, it may funnel energy away from things like cognitive functions needed for work.

This difference in temperature has also led to thermostat disputes in households around the world. A 2019 research paper called "Thermostat Wars?" diving into gender and temperature negotiations in households, concluded that "it's clear that men's preferences seem to dominate in most households." This difference in temperature preference at home has even led to the "Scandinavian sleep method," where couples sleep with separate blankets according to their own preference. This might lead to less snuggling, but improved sleep quality.

Why Women Are More "Chill"

We know that women generally feel colder in their daily lives, but are there differences in how women tolerate cold exposure as compared to men? One way researchers tried to find out is by studying if women start to shiver earlier than men. In one study, twenty men and twenty-three women were dressed in full-body suits filled with cold water (the same type Wim wore in the Michigan study). The temperature of the suits started at 75.2 degrees and was gradually decreased 1.8 to 3.6 degrees every five minutes. Shivering started at 48.2 degrees on average for men and around 52.3 degrees for women. Women reported feeling "cool" at a temperature of 64.9 degrees while men reported the same feeling at a temperature of 58.2 degrees. This demonstrates that the threshold for shivering and feeling cold is lower for women, meaning women feel colder quicker and also experience stress from the cold more rapidly. There do seem to be relevant physiological differences between men and women, including:

- BODY SIZE: Factors such as height and weight affect how quickly we lose heat. The surface area–to–mass ratio is also an essential factor in the dissipation of heat. We generate heat in proportion to our total mass and dissipate heat in proportion to our total surface area, and with more surface area relative to mass, heat escapes more quickly to the surroundings. Smaller people, like women, generally have a higher surface area–to–mass ratio, which means that women tend to produce less heat and lose heat faster through the skin than men.

- WHITE FAT: On average, women have more white fat than men. And despite what our fat-phobic world has instilled in us, this is generally beneficial for women. White fat has incredibly important functions, such as protecting the vital organs, including the uterus. White fat also acts as insulation; the more fat we have between skin and muscle, the more heat stays in. But there is also a downside to this extra layer of white fat: it can restrict blood flow to the extremities, which causes colder hands and feet in women. So: a warmer heart, but colder hands!

- BROWN FAT: When it comes to brown fat, research suggests that women have more efficient brown fat than men. Another study showed that pre-pubertal and teenage girls have more cold-induced brown fat than their male counterparts. Research comparing brown fat in adult men and women is contradictory or nonconclusive, and we're not sure how this affects the way women and men experience the cold, but we're learning more all the time.

- MUSCLE MASS: Women have lower muscle mass on average, and since muscles speed up metabolism, this means a lower metabolic rate and less heat production. That said, research shows that women actually display more efficient use of their intercostal muscles and since these muscles are also involved in utilizing glucose to produce heat, this may give them an advantage in some ways against the cold, although more research needs to be done to say for sure.

- HEART SIZE: Men tend to have more muscle mass, and that includes the size of the heart, which is the muscle that keeps the cardiovascular system running. This, along with bigger blood vessels, may allow men to pump blood more easily. It could also lead to stronger circulatory function in general, which means the core body temperature is less easily compromised.

- HORMONAL FLUCTUATIONS: Female hormones, and the way they fluctuate throughout the month during the reproductive years, influence the way women experience temperature. Women tend to have a core body temperature between 97.5 and 98 degrees, with lower temperatures during the follicular phase, or the first part of the menstrual cycle. In the follicular phase, estrogen rises and progesterone is lower, which leads to vasodilation, allowing warm blood to flow through the body more easily. The rising estrogen in this phase tends to help with heat loss. In the second phase of this cycle, the luteal phase, progesterone takes the lead, causing vasoconstriction and the preservation of heat to the point where core temperature increases by 0.9 degrees. During this phase, shivering starts earlier than in other phases; we feel colder, and we tend to dress warmer. During menstruation, we shed blood, and this can deplete iron, which can lead to a loss of energy and body heat. Because of this, going into the cold may be more challenging depending on where you are in your cycle. But if we understand how our hormones and cycles affect our temperature, we can use this knowledge to our advantage to prepare for cold exposure and increase its benefits.

BBT: TRACKING WHEN YOU ARE "IN HEAT": Did you know that your basal body temperature (BBT) can be used to track your fertility during the month? Because our body temperature changes with our hormonal fluctuations, we can track how fertile we are by measuring it. BBT increases during ovulation (when we are "in heat"), and you can measure the temperature orally or rectally. For decades, women have used the BTT method to track their fertility cycle and know when they can have sex without getting pregnant. Research has also confirmed that temperature is an accurate metric to measure the cycle phase of females. In fact, apps that use an algorithm to predict your fertility using daily temperature readings have been approved as birth control in many countries, with 93 percent efficacy with typical use and 98 percent efficacy with perfect use. Interestingly, taking hormone birth control can affect female hormones in a way that raises body temperature, leading to increased sensitivity to the cold.

Women can experience the cold differently from men, and that is an important consideration when developing a Wim Hof Method practice. The WHM is more than just turning the shower to cold or dunking in an ice bath. It's about proper mental and physical preparation that maximizes both your safety and the benefits you get.

THE 3 PHASES OF COLD EXPOSURE

If a person enters extreme cold unprepared—such as if they fall through the ice at a lake or out of a boat in the winter—they will experience something called cold shock. The immediate cooling of the skin sends signals to the brain of extreme cold detection and pain. They will then gasp for air and start hyperventilating. Their heart rate and blood pressure shoot up as their body scrambles to maintain their core body temperature. Cold shock can cause confusion and disorientation, and this massively increases the chance of swallowing a big mouthful of water. Cold shock is the leading cause of drowning, and clearly highlights how powerful the cold can be. With the WHM, we learn to deal with this initial cold shock in a controlled setting. This is also why we first properly prepare people mentally and physically, using breathing exercises to prime the mind and body. We advise to build up to ice baths slowly, starting by ending our shower briefly with cold and extending the duration of cold exposure progressively. With gradual cold exposure, we are staying safe, and we are arming ourselves to adapt mentally and physically to the extreme cold. Just like any new experience, it is essential that it is a pleasant experience to spark the right neural circuitry, to keep you coming back. This is why we always say that the first ice bath is the most important and we do recommend it be done in a proper WHM workshop. This is also why we break down the WHM cold exposure exercise into three phases. As we like to say: "The ice bath begins before we even go in."

Before

With the WHM, we prepare physically and mentally for cold exposure. Before we even think about getting into the cold, we prepare our bodies by performing the WHM breathing exercises. We start these anywhere between a couple of hours to twenty minutes before we enter the cold. This increases our pain tolerance by releasing adrenaline and switching off pain receptors, which benefits us greatly when we enter the ice bath.

Next, we establish a healthy mindset to take on the cold. For many women, the moment before an ice bath is fraught with anxiety. In this case, it's great to take a moment to close your eyes and first visualize going into the ice bath successfully. Then, we recommend setting a strong intention. Is there a limiting belief or fear you want to shatter, or a goal you have for yourself you want to reach? The ice bath can serve as an amazing metaphor for anything in your life you would like to conquer. You can decide on a mantra to repeat, such as "I am in control" or "I've got this." Just before entering, we recommend tapping a little cold water on your shoulders and neck (not coincidentally, this is near where the vagus nerve is) to get acquainted with the cold. Then take a last moment to relax the shoulders and neck and put yourself in the zone.

During

The moment you are in the ice bath, the mental exercise continues. Your body responds instantly by entering a sympathetic state, signaling loudly: "Get me the heck out of here!" The first thirty to sixty seconds are usually the hardest. When you decide mentally to stay in the cold, you are overriding the conditioned response to stay within your comfort zone. We recommend focusing on taking long out-breaths to help regulate your nervous system, which helps accelerate the adaptation process by activating your vagus nerve to bring you out of fight or flight. During these harsh moments you can focus on your intention or repeat any mantra that you like, such as "relax, nothing is under control," or "be comfortable in the uncomfortable."

After you get to the other side of the initial phase of extreme discomfort, the body starts to understand that the mind has decided to stay in the cold. With that realization, it begins to adapt and relax into the stress of the cold. Your heart rate will start to calm, and the extreme sensation or pain of the cold on your skin will ease. Your body will reward you with hormones like noradrenaline, dopamine, and beta-endorphins. These hormones act as anesthesia against the cold, helping you adapt and giving you a sense of exhilaration and well-being. For many women, this is when the emotions come out. In our trainings, we celebrate any emotions that surface—letting them go can be extremely liberating.

Isabelle: I started cold showers at around age fourteen. The first time I did an ice bath I was twenty-five. It was at one of the events we organized. I first put my hands inside for a minute, and I was shocked! It hurt me so much, and I wondered how the hell my father could stand that feeling for more than one hour! It was only when I went in and overcame the initial shock that I understood why my father was always in the cold water. It gave me such an exhilarating feeling afterward. I felt on top of the world! For me, the cold is like coffee in the morning—a quick way to feel centered and energized. Especially when I am doing it outside, I completely submerse myself in nature, leaving me with a feeling of oneness.

If you stay in the cold a little bit longer, it feels like the mind and body make a pact. This is where the magic happens. When you can release the controlling mind and let the body do the work, you allow your body to activate its primal mechanisms, which are expertly designed to protect you. Once you feel comfortable in the uncomfortable, the work has been done. You override your stress response. It's not a competition for who can stay in the cold the longest; it's about training your mindset in the cold. It's about how much you can let go mentally, connect physically, let the body do the work, and accept the difficulty of sitting in the ice bath.

After

The third step starts when we exit the cold. When you come out, you'll notice that the internal noise is gone, and you feel centered and more in tune with the world around you. It's crucial to stay focused and connected with your body directly after the ice bath. If you go in for too long and don't warm up properly, you can experience something called an after drop, making you feeling shaky and loopy. This occurs when the warm blood from your core is needed to warm up the body parts that cooled down in the cold. The muscles, fat, and blood outside your core cool off during cold exposure and continue to cool off until you've warmed up. The process of heating those up takes it away from your core, which causes a sudden drop in temperature. Since the core body temperature cannot be compromised, this temperature drop jump-starts the body's quickest response for heat production in order to survive: shivering. A common first-timers' mistake is to stay in the cold too long. Once the body adapts to the cold, you feel you can stay in for longer, but the temperature in your arms and legs, both muscle and fat, will keep getting lower and lower. This can make the after drop an extremely uncomfortable experience and is why it's important to ease into cold exposure—we recommend that beginners only stay in the cold for a maximum of two to three minutes—bring a buddy, and always pay attention to your body. If you start to shiver, which is likely to happen at the beginning of your training but decreases with repeat training, your job is to focus and tell your body that it is safe. When people lose their focus in extreme cold conditions, uncontrollable shivering kicks in immediately. One second of mental distraction and your body seems to say, "You are not here with me anymore, so I have to take over." Controlling your shivering is a sign not only of physical adaptation, but of an improved mind-body connection. This leads to greater mental control over your physiology.

To prevent the after drop and shivering once you exit the ice bath, we recommend warming up from within using "Horsestance." This activates the core muscles and the leg muscles, which we call the "big heaters" because they are the biggest muscles in the body. Horsestance is essentially a deep wide-legged squat, with the feet turned out, a bit like how a samurai or sumo wrestler stands when they are ready for action. Stay completely focused on your body and tell it, "I'm here with you." Then, activate the muscles further by slowly moving the upper body side to side, engaging the intercostal muscles and the diaphragm. When you do this, you are heating up from the inside, and this heat will be used to warm up the cooler parts of the body. Take the time to really warm up from the inside. After about five minutes of this—it may take more time or less depending on how long you were in the cold—the extremities will warm up and your body temperature will equalize. This way of heating up involves activating important muscles but also focusing the mind; it's like training the muscle that connects the mind and body. And like any training, practice makes perfect. During our Icewomen dips we also encourage dancing after a few minutes of focused horsestance.

COLD CONDITIONING

Doing an ice bath for the first time is like doing two exercises in one. There's the ice bath itself, which is something new, but there's also the task of doing something completely out of your comfort zone. The second time you enter freezing water will already be easier, as you will understand the cold better and how you react to it.

After decades of involvement in cold exposure practices, we have consistently observed that the more you engage in cold exposure, the better your body adapts to it. This is due to improvements in cardiovascular function, a reduced sympathetic response, enhanced glucose sensitivity, increased brown fat activation, and the training of muscles to boost metabolic activity. One study on women showed that after twelve weeks of cold exposure three times a week, noradrenaline levels were consistent (increasing two- to threefold after twenty seconds of cold exposure in water 32 to 35.6 degrees), but cortisol levels were significantly lower in week twelve than in week one, indicating a lowered "stress" response. Other research showed that cold exposure to a 50-degree room for two hours every day led to a decrease in sympathetic response and an increase in parasympathetic activity over ten days. This means a more relaxed nervous system over time with repeated cold exposure! Finally, one study showed that it takes an average of six ice dips to reduce the cold water shock by 50 percent when doing ice water swimming. When using the WHM breathing and mindset techniques, you can expect to adapt even faster. With proper training, beginners often complete the second ice bath immersion cool as a cucumber.

You will adapt to the extreme cold the more you do it, but the opposite is also true: you have to use it, or you will lose it! Research into female Korean free divers called Haenyeo (similar to the Japanese Ama) confirms this. During the nineteenth century, 22 percent of all Korean women on Jeju Island were "seawomen," diving in deep, cold waters (between 55.4 and 57.2 degrees in the winter) while dressed in only thin cotton bathing suits. These women had a great tolerance toward cold water, but when they stopped their cold water practices, their cold adaptation disappeared. Continuous conditioning to cold is therefore essential to maintain the ability to deal with cold.

DO YOUR GENES AFFECT YOUR RESILIENCE TO THE COLD? Many people from mostly Latin American, African, and Middle Eastern backgrounds come to Wim Hof Method trainings commenting that they are made for warm temperatures, with their argument being that their genetic makeup does not allow them to be resilient in the cold. And it is true that genetics make a difference in how they handle the cold. However, mindset and mental conditioning are far more important. Research on various people and cultures around the world shows that our bodies change and adapt to the cold just the same.

HOW TO CHILL: COLD EXPOSURE FOR WOMEN

Although we have guidelines and best practices, there are no dogmatic WHM rules about the best way to do cold exposure: each physiology is different. Our research and experience have allowed us to create a framework that allows you to explore what works for you since, as we know, factors such as height, weight, and prior experience affect how we experience the cold. This is in line with a guiding principle within the WHM: "Feeling is understanding."

For women this is even more important, as we are more sensitive to stress and have additional hormonal factors that influence the cold exposure. Regardless of type of cold exposure, temperature, and duration, cold exposure should always be done in tune with your body, as each person has a different physiology. We also like to say: "The average is not the individual, and the individual is not the average."

The beauty of the cold is that it puts you directly in contact with your body, so you will be given important cues throughout the experience. Your body will tell you when you can push just a little further, and it will tell you when you should be done for the day. Through practicing the WHM, this awareness of the body, which we call "interoceptive focus," increases as well. This will strengthen your ability to use your body's compass when training with the cold.

Cold exposure should be tailored to one's capability and gradually built up, but it's helpful to start with some general parameters and guidelines for working with the cold.

Types of Cold Exposure

There are many ways to work with the cold. You could take a cold shower, try an ice bath, swim in the winter waters, or simply turn down the thermostat in your home. You might be wondering why you must involve water at all: Isn't a wintry walk or hike enough to get the same effects? One thing to consider is that water's thermal conductance is about twenty-five times greater than that of air. In cold water, you lose heat two to five times more quickly than when you expose yourself to cold air at the same temperature. During our winter expeditions, we lead groups of participants to a freezing-cold mountain, hiking at minus 23 degrees in shorts and a sports bra for multiple hours. This would never be possible in water. This also explains why cryotherapy chambers can be set far colder than an ice bath. While water acts as a conductor, air acts as an insulator, which means it's not as efficient. This is why we mostly recommend water-based cold exposure practice, starting with:

- COLD SHOWER: We always recommend starting your cold exposure practice with a cold shower since they are the most accessible way to practice daily. Not everyone will have an ice bath, waterfall, or cold river in their backyard, but nearly everybody does have a shower! You can start by simply ending your warm shower with ten seconds of cold, and gradually build up to two minutes or more of cold at the end. Normally, we recommend doing this in the morning to energize your body, like a strong cup of coffee. Other optimal times include before a workout, as the release of noradrenaline mobilizes the body and muscles. You can even target your armpits as they are warmer and contain important sweat glands and will increase the energy boost. For many people, a cold shower works wonderfully as a stress reset any time of day. We recommend a cold shower daily, which is easy since most of us shower every day anyway. As our dad always says: "A cold shower a day keeps the doctor away." Of course, you can skip a day or a few when your body doesn't feel like it—always listen to your body. If you live in a warm place, like Dubai or Australia, your shower might not get extremely cold even on the coldest setting. But rest assured that contrast is important and the blue knob in these countries will still feel quite cold when you're used to a warm, sunny environment.

- THE ICE BATH: It's usually the ice bath people want to conquer when coming to a Wim Hof Method workshop. As it's also the most intense form of cold exposure, the ice bath is the best tool for building up your mental resilience and the quickest way to increase your ability to adapt to stress. To overcome your stress response and relax into the cold, stay in for two to three minutes. This is just enough to get out of the sympathetic state and relax in the stress, and a great booster for your body. You can look up ice bathing in your area, or create one in your own bathtub or backyard.

- NATURAL COLD WATER SWIMMING: Even better than cold showers or ice baths are natural bodies of cold water, including waterfalls, ponds, creeks, rivers, lakes, and oceans. Cold water swimming in nature is like medicine. There's something about a natural body of water that nothing else can beat. This may be because being in nature has a positive impact on mental health, as it activates the parasympathetic nervous system. Entering this type of water, you feel like you become one with nature. It washes away your worries, centers you, and brings you clarity. In Gerald Pollack's book *The Fourth Phase of Water*, he talks about how objects in cold water experience a powerful negative charge, which acts like a battery charging the object. When you swim in cold natural water, you are the object and receive this charge. Most toxins, harmful chemicals, and even cell phones and computers have a positive electrical charge, which can have a negative impact on our health, mood, and energy levels. Negative ions can be found in abundance in natural environments, such as mountains, oceans, forests, and waterfalls, and during storms and rain (and even to a small degree a simple cold shower, even in an apartment in a bustling city!).

- STILL VERSUS RUNNING WATER: Interestingly, there is a big difference between running water and still water. When we're sitting still in an ice bath, we create a layer of heat just around our bodies. But when we're in running cold water, such as a waterfall or a river, this layer of heat is constantly washed away. If you want to challenge yourself in an ice bath, move your arms, legs, and hands. You can instantly feel the difference.
- COLD EXPOSURE GADGETS: Nowadays, more devices are coming on the market to help us chill, such as cold packs, cold suits, facial chillers, and portable ice baths. Our advice is to keep it simple: end your showers with cold, go outside in shorts and a T-shirt even when it's cold, and even try to avoid bundling up with a scarf and hat on the first cool day of winter. Even a slight decrease in temperature can lead to the activation of heat-generating pathways and provide mood and health benefits.

Cold exposure should always be done to fit your needs. And although our mantra is to do the type, duration, and form that suit you, we have specific protocols at the end of this chapter, guidelines on how to plan around your cycle in Chapter 10, and a 30-Day Icewoman Challenge for those who need a little structure to get them started in the final chapter. Protocols and rules are only a starting point, and can be abandoned once you strengthen your mind-body connection and interoceptive focus.

9 Women-Centric Tips for Cold Exposure

After decades of practice, research, and most of all, experience in this field, here are our best tips for women experimenting with cold exposure.

1. DON'T PUSH IT: Even more for women than men, it is extremely important not to go beyond your limits with your cold practice. Go slowly and stay in touch with your body to understand your comfort zone and to be able to push your limits in a gentle way. Focus on creating a feeling of safety first, which will then allow you to explore your boundaries. As women we can often feel disconnected from our bodies, which can cause us to push ourselves when we actually need to rest.

2. CONNECT WITH OTHER WOMEN: The tend-and-befriend reaction teaches us that as women, we have a deep urge for social connection and acceptance. Social connection also boosts oxytocin, a hormone women need to offset the effect of the stress hormone cortisol. Without sacrificing your own individual journey, connect with other women through your cold exposure training. Even better, try to enlist the support of someone who is well practiced in cold exposure. It's nice to know that others have your back.

3. TRUST YOUR BODY'S ABILITY TO DO THE WORK: Remember that your body is built to deal with the impact of a two-minute ice bath. And your physiological processes will kick in automatically—no conscious or anxious thoughts required. The only thing you must focus on is relaxing mentally and allowing your body to do the work.

4. ALLOW YOURSELF TO FEEL THE EMOTIONS THAT ARISE: Crying is absolutely normal. Emotions are beautiful; let them go. The cold is a huge form of stress, and we often get emotional in response; it's simply that those feelings were ready to be released. Many of us hold on to our emotions for dear life, when it's natural and healthy to let them go.

5. ADJUST YOUR PRACTICE TO YOUR MENSTRUAL CYCLE: Track where you are in your cycle and adjust your cold practice routine. For example, when it's your first time doing an ice bath, do it around the end of your follicular phase (day ten to twelve after your menstruation started, when estrogen is at its highest level). For more information on this, go to Chapter 10.

6. PROTECT THE HANDS AND FEET: As we learned, women have colder hands and feet. It's okay to put your fingers outside the ice bath. Put your hands in a prayer position with the fingers out of the water or get some gloves for your hands and water shoes for your feet when going out into nature. You can also practice the cold hand and feet exercise on pages 83–84 a few times a week.

7. GET HELP WARMING UP: If you still feel cold an hour after cold exposure, take a warm shower. There's no need to feel cold for the whole day! If you feel cold hours after your cold exposure, it's also a sign you were overdoing it.

8. BE AWARE OF YOUR POSTURE: This will boost your confidence and have a positive impact on your physiology. Practice the Power Woman Pose (as described in the following Cold Water Protocols for Women).

9. TREAT YOURSELF: Buy yourself a nice bathing suit or bikini, and a beautiful robe, as research says: if you feel hot, you'll feel less cold!

COLD WATER PROTOCOLS FOR WOMEN

The cold is a powerful force, and extreme cold can shock our bodies. It is therefore important to practice responsibly and be prepared. It is vital to slowly and gradually build up cold training. Never force your cold training. People with cardiovascular issues, or any other severe health conditions, should always consult a medical professional before starting the Wim Hof Method.

The first step is to understand what the cold does to the body and understand your boundaries with it. Your body and mind need time to adapt to the cold, so start with simply ending your showers with cold water in the comfort of your home. If you decide to take the next step with ice baths or nature dips, always bring a buddy. When practicing in a group, keep an eye on others. Someone who appears completely fine getting out of the water may still need attention ten minutes later.

Protocol 1: The Ice Bath Protocol

A crucial cold exposure element is having the right mindset and mental state. The ice bath experience doesn't begin when you're in the water—it starts beforehand. Your posture sends signals to your mind: Are we safe, or should we be afraid? By standing tall and strong, you signal to your body and mind that you're prepared to face the challenge ahead. You communicate that you're in control. The "power pose" is known to reduce cortisol, which is why we recommend it to the women in our workshops before they enter the ice bath. Your initial state of mind matters! So, like Wonder Woman, stand up straight with your hands on your hips or by your sides and a relaxed neck and shoulders. Stand tall, confident, and proud—as if you're ready to take on the world.

How to do it:

1. Start by setting your intention: Why are you taking the ice bath? Focus your mind.

2. Step into the Power Woman Pose (stand confidently—you've got this!).

3. Focus on your breath.

4. Prepare by splashing cold water on your neck, shoulders, and arms to get accustomed to the cold.

5. Return to your Power Woman Pose and reconnect with your intention or mantra (e.g., "feeling comfortable in the uncomfortable," "I've got this," or "relax, nothing is under control").

6. When you feel ready, step into the ice bath with a strong mindset.

7. Submerge your full body on a long exhale with your shoulders down and relaxed. The quicker and more fully submerged your whole body is, the quicker you adapt. Place your hands on your thighs or under your armpits, or put them in prayer position, with your fingers slightly outside the water.

8. Keep your focus on your breath, slowly returning it to normal while extending your exhales.

9. Connect with your body, embrace the cold like a warm friend, and release resistance whenever you feel it mentally or physically.

10. Stay until you feel a shift in both body and mind, having overcome your initial stress response. For beginners, stay in the ice bath for a maximum of two to three minutes. If you're more advanced, you can gradually add more time until you find your ideal duration.

Protocol 2: Cold/Hot Shower Protocol

How to do it:

1. Prepare your mind before your cold shower. The morning is the best time, as starting your day with a challenge sets the tone. By choosing to take that cold shower, you defeat your inner saboteur right away.

2.   At the end of your warm shower, turn the water to cold.

3.   Stand so the water hits your neck and shoulders, letting it run over your entire body. Avoid having it hit your head, except if you really feel you want to. Move around to ensure maximum exposure, and for an extra challenge, rinse under your armpits.

4.   Do not do breathing exercises while standing in the shower as they can make you feel lightheaded and you don't want to fall.

5.   Start with fifteen seconds of cold exposure, gradually increasing it each day to one to two minutes.

6.   Switch the water back to warm, rinsing your entire body for two minutes.

7.   Alternate between cold and warm water for up to two minutes each, repeating this cycle two to three times. Always end with cold water to close your pores and allow your veins to relax naturally.

8.   Enjoy the invigorating sensation!

Laura: I have been doing cold showers since I was eleven, but I have always done it alternating with warm water. This eased my practice and has always made me want to go back to it no matter what the temperature is during the year, or where I am in my cycle. I believe this type of practice is a better fit for ladies since it can be done during the whole of a woman's cycle, without anything feeling too intense. Personally, I also think the temperature contrast between warm and cold makes this the most invigorating way to do a cold shower!

Protocol 3: Warmer Hands and Feet

Women have colder hands and feet, and how cold we feel depends greatly on the temperature of the extremities. This exercise is a great way to train for warmer hands and feet and you will also feel invigorated afterward! Do this exercise a couple of times per week.

How to do it:

1. Fill a bucket with two-thirds water and one-third ice.
2. Place your hands and/or feet in the water and focus on your breath. Accept whatever sensations arise in that moment.
3. After two to five minutes, remove your hands and/or feet from the water.
4. Warm them up by shaking or flapping them quickly to encourage blood flow.
5. Repeat steps 2 to 4, two to three times.

Protocol 4: Warm Up the Hands After Cold Exposure

After cold exposure, like a freezing nature swim, the hands can feel extremely cold and numb. The following exercise helps Isabelle feel amazing after extreme cold exposure:

How to do it:

1. Take a deep breath in and hold it.
2. Make your hands into a fist.
3. Activate the muscles in the hands and give them a good strong press.
4. With the outbreath, let go and simultaneously relax the hands.
5. Repeat steps 1 to 4 until you feel the heat returning to the hands and fingers.

After many years of leading thousands of women through their first cold exposure experience, what is clear to us is that while women might be more anxious before submerging themselves in the cold, they are perfectly equipped to adapt to the cold and reap all of its benefits. Like the Ama and their pearls, the cold gives us the opportunity to become stronger, more resilient, healthier, and happier. With the help of the Wim Hof Method, women transform from worriers into warriors.

5

A DEEP EXHALE: WOMEN AND BREATH

"Control your breath, control your life force."

Most women attending our workshops come for the thrill of the ice bath (and of course, the photo!). And yet they almost always depart most profoundly impacted by the breathing exercises. A single session of WHM breathing takes you on a profound journey, connecting you deeply with your heart, unleashing a spectrum of emotions and releasing tension and stress from your body and mind. You leave feeling more alive, balanced, and emotionally strong. The cold gets us more in touch with our bodies, but the breathing works to get us out of our heads. You only have to experience it once to understand the immense power of the breath.

The breath is our most powerful instrument, a tool that accompanies us not just through every phase of life but every moment of it. The breath is an energizer and a decompressor; it makes you stop and go, panic or relax, and rush or slow down. As we always say in our trainings: control your breath and you control your life force.

The breath has the power to give women what they desperately need to gain more energy, overcome stressors, and regulate their internal state. And yet we often overlook this incredible resource within us, taking it for granted. In this chapter, you will learn that the simple inhales and exhales you take every day are more than meets the eye.

INHALE AND EXHALE: THE JOURNEY OF THE BREATH

When we enter the world, our first act is to inhale and then exhale, releasing a cry announcing our arrival. From that moment on, we breathe approximately twenty thousand times a day until our very last breath—our last moment on Earth. While we can survive weeks without food and days without water, we cannot endure more than a few minutes without breathing. Breathing is the most fundamental human action, vital for supplying the body with oxygen, driving energy production, and sustaining all our bodily processes. Every organ and cell relies on the breath to function.

AN ANCIENT PERSPECTIVE ON THE BREATH AND BREATH PRACTICES:
Ancient cultures saw the breath not only as the physical air taken into the lungs but also as a life force. The term "breath" is often translated to mean "spirit" or "soul." In Latin, "spiritus" refers both to the act of breathing and to "spirit" or "soul." Similarly, the Greek word "pneuma" means both "air/breath" and "spirit" or "life energy," reflecting the Greeks' belief in the connection between breath, mind, and spirit. In ancient Indian philosophy, "prana" translates to "breath" and "air," but also signifies the "sacred essence of life." In China, "chi" denotes both the breath and the "universal and cosmic energy of life."

The main job of the respiratory system is to drive the exchange of oxygen and carbon dioxide between our bodies and our environment. When we breathe in, it takes about one minute for the air we've inhaled to make a complete journey through the body. In this minute, millions of processes take place. Air goes into our lungs and travels through the main bronchial tubes to microscopic air sacs called alveoli, where oxygen and carbon dioxide are exchanged. The alveoli are surrounded by red blood cells, which have the important job of carrying the oxygen in the air we've inhaled so it can enter the bloodstream. After the exchange, the heart pumps the newly oxygenated blood around the body to tissues and organs until it finds cells in need of oxygen. An average adult woman has about 28 trillion hungry cells that feed themselves with oxygen and, in return, unload carbon dioxide, which the red blood cells carry back to the lungs to be exhaled into the environment. While we might think we breathe in pure oxygen, air is about 78 percent nitrogen, 21 percent oxygen, and 1 percent other gases, including 0.4 percent carbon dioxide. When we exhale, the air consists of around 4 percent carbon dioxide, 17 percent unused oxygen, 78 percent nitrogen, and 1 percent other gases. This incredible exchange of life force with our environment even changes the appearance of our blood, with oxygen-rich blood looking bright red while blood carrying carbon dioxide appears blue.

This process occurs every moment we're alive. You might wonder why our cells require this much oxygen. The reason is simple: energy. Our cells need oxygen to produce the energy that keeps us living, loving, and healthy. When oxygen enters the body's cells, it combines with glucose to break down and produce a molecule called adenosine triphosphate (ATP). This process, called cellular respiration, is what produces the carbon dioxide the body has to then exhale.

ATP is essentially our fuel to live, storing and transporting energy within cells. Like batteries powering a flashlight or gas powering a car, ATP is the energy currency required for muscle movement, nutrient transfer, waste removal, and nerve signal transmission. The breakdown of glucose and oxygen into ATP occurs in the 1,000 to 2,500 mitochondria—known as "energy factories"—we have in each cell. The process of cellular respiration can occur without oxygen in some cases, but it is much less efficient, with eighteen times less ATP produced per molecule of glucose. Oxygen is no doubt a critical factor in the body's overall energy production. And with women reporting higher levels of fatigue than men, it's especially important for us to understand the role the breath can play in our energy levels. Perhaps oxygen is that vital life force that you have been missing!

WHM BREATHING FOR ENDURANCE TRAINING: Without enough oxygen, cellular respiration will be much less efficient and can also result in a buildup of waste products, like lactic acid. If you're an athlete, you know that lactic acid is what's responsible for the burning sensation, fatigue, and "hitting a wall" during a workout or training. Interestingly, the results of one study showed that WHM breathing activates the Cori cycle, which impacts the body's ability to recycle lactic acid byproducts back to glucose, which can then be used again to produce more ATP—a sort of fuel recycling! This indicates breathing exercises may have a positive effect on endurance training, preventing lactic acid buildup. I (Laura) credit the breath for helping me complete a marathon easily and without soreness. When I was running and felt low on energy, I would breathe in a little bit more air than I thought necessary. The breath has an incredible power to rebalance, restore, and maintain your energy levels!

We need to breathe to survive and fuel our cells, but how we breathe may be even more important for our health. How we breathe not only influences our physiology and energy production, but also our state of being and our emotions.

THE BREATH: THE REMOTE CONTROL OF THE NERVOUS SYSTEM

Breathing "practices" or "breathwork" have gained significant meaning and popularity in the Western world in recent years, but Eastern traditions have recognized the power of the breath for thousands of years. Some of the earliest examples of manipulating the breath for meditative relaxation, self-healing, emotion regulation, and spiritual connection date back to 5000 BCE in ancient India. Extraordinary yogis throughout history could slow down their heart rate at will, which was seen as impossible for the laywoman. But now we know that we can all use our breath to do this and much more.

The breath is fascinating in that it is the only part of our nervous system that is automatic—we don't have to consciously remember to breathe at all hours of the day—but that we can also consciously influence. With that understanding, the breath becomes the gateway to willfully take the reins over the autonomic nervous system and all the systems it directly or indirectly regulates, such as your cardiovascular, digestion, and hormonal system.

Your internal state and your breath are intrinsically linked, and you can assess which state someone is in simply by observing their breathing. When you watch a frequent meditator, like a monk, for example, you might notice the way they breathe calmly, softly, slowly, and through the nose as they sit almost motionless. They are clearly in a state of peace and relaxation, and appear joyful. Comparatively, when a person is angry or stressed, their breath becomes shallow, quick, and jagged.

Our emotions influence our breathing pattern, but this connection is a two-way street. We can also change our breathing to evoke a specific internal state. Slow, deep breathing into the belly will activate your parasympathetic nervous system and vagus nerve, promoting a state of relaxation and ease. Fast and short breaths through the mouth

A SIGH OF RELIEF: A quick way to release stress using the breath is through three simple sighs, and this is also the way I (Laura) start any WHM breathing session. I have everyone do three sighs with the aim of relaxing the mind, releasing stored tension, and grounding themselves in the moment. This great little nugget of an exercise has been celebrated by the likes of Andrew Huberman, and many yoga classes start this way. You might have already used the sigh unconsciously when you were frustrated, felt bored, needed to blow off steam, or felt in a state of depression. It's a way to stimulate the vagus nerve and regulate quickly, and it helps us to feel safe, relaxed, and content.

activate the sympathetic nervous system, which causes our heart rate to accelerate and our blood pressure to rise. This can be helpful in some circumstances—for example, when you need to accomplish a big task, a tough workout, or when in need of some extra energy—but is not ideal for everyday breathing.

Unfortunately, many of us have gotten into a habit of breathing in a way that activates the sympathetic nervous system all the time. Most of the time, this dysfunctional breathing pattern is caused by stress. When we've been in fight-or-flight mode regularly, our breathing pattern will match this mode as well, with our breathing mechanics and muscles adapting to this. In our WHM retreats, we often help participants identify their baseline breathing patterns. Oftentimes it's a massive "Aha!" moment when women realize they've been breathing in a way that promotes the cycle of stress for years or even decades on end.

Breath Assessment: Measuring Your Baseline

This assessment is a great way to find out if your baseline breathing pattern is promoting stress or relaxation. Do this assessment a couple of times before making any firm conclusions. To do it, sit or lie down, relax, and just take a moment to become aware of your breathing. Ask yourself the following questions:

1. Are you breathing through your nose or mouth?
2. Is your spine straight or bent slightly forward? Are your chest and shoulders open and expanded or closed and hunched?
3. Put one hand on your belly and one on your chest. With the inhale, is your chest expanding or is your belly expanding?
4. Look at a clock or set a timer on your phone. How many breaths are you taking per minute?

If you find you take fewer than twelve breaths per minute, through the nose, with an open posture, and your belly expands on the inhale, then your regular breathing pattern is already pretty optimal. If you take more than twelve breaths per minute, breathe through the mouth, have a closed posture, or notice your chest expands on the inbreath, then it's a sign you've got some relearning to do.

The 4 Fundamentals of Healthy Breathing

When you practice WHM breathing, your breathing mechanics and patterns will start to change, and these four things will begin to happen automatically, subconsciously, and naturally, which indicates a calm and content state. Your body knows best and will realign itself naturally through practicing the method, creating a more healthy everyday breathing pattern. The difference between the WHM method and many other modules that require rigorous training and conscious effort is that the method allows our bodies to rearrange themselves subconsciously, with little effort. You simply have to do fifteen to twenty minutes of WHM breathing daily.

1. **Open posture**

   Our posture influences our breathing, and our breathing influences our posture. It's a simple fact that we can breathe more deeply when our head and shoulders are in line with the rest of the body, and we have a straight back and open chest and shoulders. When someone is at a WHM workshop, we can almost immediately tell if their breathing patterns will need to be addressed based on their posture. When a person looks stiff, especially in their shoulders and neck, and their head also tends to be a bit more forward, it's a telltale sign of unhealthy breathing patterns.

2. **Slow down**

   The urge to breathe too much and too fast is usually due to stress and can decrease your tolerance to carbon dioxide over time, leading to an urge to keep breathing more than is necessary. Long exhales are one of the principles we teach our students because they naturally slow down the breathing. By deepening your breath and focusing on longer exhales (sometimes even doubling the length of the exhale), you stimulate the vagus nerve and parasympathetic nervous system and desensitize your chemoreceptors to tolerate higher levels of carbon dioxide, which means you breathe a little less. Occasionally, we also tell participants to use humming or the word "om" when we see they are having difficulty staying in the ice bath. These practices activate our vagus nerve, help us get in the zone, open up the veins fifteen- to twentyfold, and help us relax.

3. **Breathe deeply into the belly**

   If you noticed your chest expanding on your inhale during the breathing assessment, this one is for you. As the biggest breathing muscle, our diaphragm is an extremely important part of the respiratory system. Sometimes referred to as our "second heart," it moves down during inhalation, opening the rib cage and pushing the organs down to make space for the lungs to expand. To properly activate your diaphragm, the belly should expand on the inhale. Begin by breathing into the belly and abdominal area, allowing it to expand, and then let the breath naturally fill the chest. When we fully engage the diaphragm during our inhale, we:

- Create more space for the lungs to expand (The surface area of healthy lungs can expand to as big as three-quarters of a tennis court!)
- Activate the vagus nerve and the parasympathetic nervous system
- Promote more efficient oxygen uptake
- Activate the pelvic floor (more on this later in the chapter)

4. **Inhale through the nose**

   In nine out of ten WHM workshops, we get the question: Does it matter if I breathe in through my nose or mouth? In relation to the fifteen-to-twenty-minute WHM breathing exercises, it doesn't matter (as Wim always says: "Breathe through any hole you have!"). Whatever it takes for you to fully and actively inhale. But for everyday breathing, you should be breathing through the nose. Nose breathing is linked to deeper breathing and engages the diaphragm and activates the parasympathetic nervous system. Nose breathing also releases a molecule called nitric oxide (NO), which opens up your veins and allows 20 percent more oxygen in, according to one study. Nose breathing also helps capture pathogens before they enter the body past your nose hairs, and your nasal passages work to moisturize the air, which is better for your lungs.

While there are more detailed protocols later in this chapter, it's important to know how to put these four fundamentals into practice right away. Do this brief exercise to guide you in retraining your breath:

1. Before starting, take a moment to assess your body. Notice how you feel and any areas of tension or stress. Focus on these areas with your breath, taking deep inhales and relaxed exhales.

2. First, consciously follow your breath and focus on breathing through the nose on the inhale and exhaling through the mouth. Spend a few breaths on this step.

3. Next, put one hand on your belly and one on your chest. With the inhale, breathe deeper into your belly. Focus on the belly expanding on the inhale, instead of the chest rising on the inhale. *Tip:* If you're struggling with this, sometimes it's easier to put both hands on the sides of your belly and breathe into both hands.

4. Finally, slow down your breathing, paying attention to deepening each breath. Slow down to ten breaths or fewer (ideally six!) per minute.

5. Keep in mind, it may take some time to relearn healthy and relaxed breathing patterns. Be patient with yourself!

The power of the breath is something we carry within us like a potent treasure, ready to be unleashed to transform our state of being at any time. Soon we'll explore the specifics of WHM breathwork, but first, it's important to recognize that, like cold exposure, women have unique considerations when it comes to breathing.

WOMEN AND THE BREATH

Research tells us that breathing requires more energy from women than men. Female anatomy, hormonal fluctuations, and pregnancy-related changes are just a few factors that influence how efficiently women breathe and, in turn, how we must approach breathwork.

- BREATHING RATE: Research shows that women have a higher breathing rate and move less air with each breath compared to men. This can affect how efficiently women breathe and supply the body with oxygen. This is especially true during exercise; the same research shows that women's breathing muscles require more oxygen, causing other muscles to get less, which may affect endurance or athletic performance.
- AIRWAYS AND LUNGS: Women generally have narrower airway passages than men, resulting in increased airway resistance. Women also tend to have a slightly different lung shape and smaller lungs and lung capacity than men. This means men have greater lung capacity and more alveoli to efficiently exchange oxygen and carbon dioxide.
- RIB CAGE, CHEST, AND BELLY: On average, women's rib cages are smaller and rounder. Women are also able to "open their chests" better than men, expanding them sideways instead of downward. This way of breathing allows women to make space for growing a child during pregnancy, when the growing baby displaces the lungs upward, taking up space in the belly. Evolutionarily, this adaptation may help minimize the effects of hormonal and anatomical changes during pregnancy on lung function and abdominal pressure. The expansion of the rib cage and chest may also be what allows women to use their intercostal muscles (those between the ribs) more efficiently, which gives them a leg up in heat generation, although more research is needed to say for sure.
- DIAPHRAGM: Women's anatomy allows them to breathe better during pregnancy but also predisposes us to a more stress-based type of breathing that engages the rib cage and chest instead of the diaphragm. The average male diaphragm is also 9 percent larger than the average woman's, allowing for deeper breaths. This is especially the case when seated or bent over, but is not as true when lying down.

BREATHING AND PREGNANCY: The experience of pregnancy, child-birth, and postpartum is intimately connected to the breath. With a growing belly, it can become very difficult to breathe, with 60 to 70 percent of pregnant women reporting shortness of breath, also known as "dyspnea." While giving birth, women use short puffs of air to breathe away the pain. Between contractions, we take deep breaths in through the nose and then force the air out through the mouth, using the exhale to recover, relax, and prepare the body for the next bout of pain. When it's finally time to push, the mother takes a deep breath in and holds it for dear life, using this life force to squeeze all the muscles of the body and push the baby out. And then—with the first breath in—a new life has entered the world, and is breathing all on its own for the very first time. During the postpartum period, engaging the pelvic diaphragm through breathwork can help with recovery.

- PELVIC FLOOR: Pelvic health is very important and very much connected to a healthy respiratory system. The pelvic floor consists of muscles and connective tissues holding and supporting the bladder, bowel, and sexual organs. Through the tissue (fascia), the pelvis is connected from the "floor" all the way to your nose. Pregnancy can increase the activity of the pelvic floor, which can lead to various pelvic floor issues and disorders, like incontinence. In fact, a staggering one in three women will suffer a pelvic floor disorder (PFD) in their lifetime, and this can affect our breathing mechanics, since our diaphragm can be considered the pelvic "roof." The two move in tandem; when the diaphragm moves down, the pelvic floor moves down as well, and when the diaphragm moves up, the pelvic floor moves up. This means that dysfunction in one can affect the other, but also that reestablishing the function of one can improve the other.

- FEMALE HORMONES: In the very first stage of lung development, you can already see sex differences between male and female fetuses. Sex hormones regulate lung growth, with estrogens having a stimulatory effect on lung development while androgens, like testosterone, have mainly an inhibitory effect. Estrogens also have a protective effect on the lungs, which explains why premature female babies are at lower risk for breathing difficulties. The differences don't end in babyhood, either. There is a strong connection between reproductive hormones and respiratory function. Progesterone acts as a respiratory stimulant and is one of the reasons why women breathe faster than men. Progesterone also seems to increase carbon dioxide sensitivity, which in turn can increase our breathing rate (as the desire to breathe depends on CO_2). Rising levels of progesterone in the luteal phase cause women to breathe even faster and shallower, which may explain why the symptoms of PMS are similar to the symptoms of chronic hyperventilation and symptoms like wheezing, shortness of breath, and coughing are affected by where a woman is in her cycle. It may also explain why women feel colder in this phase, as this higher breathing rate may lead to the vasoconstriction that makes women feel colder. We'll learn more about how to adapt your WHM practice to your monthly cycle, but this explains why paying extra attention to breathwork may be even more important during the luteal phase.

Certain aspects of female physiology seem to put us at a slight disadvantage when it comes to healthy breathing patterns, but after years of teaching women the WHM, we can say that it is no less life-changing for women than for men. To explain why it's so transformative, we'll dive into the biochemistry of WHM breathing.

WHM BREATHWORK: PLAYING WITH BIOCHEMISTRY

With one WHM breathing session, which consists of several rounds of active breathing and breath holds, we train the full spectrum of our nervous system: from sympathetic (active breathing) to parasympathetic (breath holds). We fully engage the nervous system through the breath, and then like a reset, bring it back to a more homeostatic baseline, moving it out of sympathetic dominance. The default baseline of our nervous system in our current lifestyle (between the sympathetic and parasympathetic) has often been conditioned in such a way that it is not close enough to the parasympathetic level, where the baseline allows for deep restorative rest. We have had many people report that after just a few rounds of WHM breathing, their whole body was more relaxed than it had been in months, or even years.

With the lifestyle many of us live today, our bodies have been conditioned to default to stressful breathing, which puts us in a more activated sympathetic nervous system. This means that our parasympathetic nervous system, which allows for deep restorative rest, is less active.

Doing the breathing exercises is like a workout where we reset our nervous system and drop our stress baseline to a more homeostatic balance point. In fact, the higher the adrenaline spike, as part of a hormetic stressor, the greater the reset of our stress baseline. Doing the Wim Hof Method breathing produces more adrenaline than in someone who is about to do their first bungee jump. All while lying on a mat. A study done on the WHM in collaboration with Queensland University that has not yet been published also showed that the resting heart rate lowered following the WHM. Just like with a big workout, breathing exercises require a big effort, but after, we feel invincible and relaxed at the same time. In one session, we shake off the stress instead of holding on to it in our bodies, just like a bunny does after evading a predator.

We are healthiest when our autonomic nervous system is able to synchronize or switch smoothly from an active state to a rest-and-recover state, depending on what the specific situation requires. Through breathing we increase the flexibility of our nervous system to adapt to any situation, from being active to deep rest. This "nervous system flexibility," as I (Laura) like to call it, lets our heart rate or cortisol levels return quickly to a normal baseline as we move through challenges more smoothly without the stress accumulating.

In 2023, we collaborated on an experiment, the results of which have not yet been published, with Dr. Henk-Jan Boele, a medical doctor and assistant professor of neuroscience at Erasmus University Medical Center who specializes in startle reflex research. Dr. Boele was particularly interested in exploring the effects of the WHM breathing techniques on this reflex.

The startle reflex is an automatic response to sudden or intense stimuli, like a loud noise or a quick movement. The reflex is a survival mechanism, rooted in our fight-or-flight response, allowing quick reaction to potential dangers. In adults, it's typically characterized by tensing muscles and blinking. The startle reflex is closely linked to the amygdala, which plays a key role in processing emotions, particularly fear. When we encounter a sudden or threatening stimulus, the amygdala quickly assesses it as a potential threat and activates the startle reflex.

The study introduced a startle reflex test to measure automatic reactions across three groups: (1) a control group, (2) experienced practitioners of the WHM breathing, and (3) participants who had just completed a WHM breathing session. The control group exhibited a typical startle response to a sudden sound, whereas both experienced WHM practitioners and participants fresh from a breathing session demonstrated a significantly reduced startle response. This suggests that the WHM, especially the breathing exercise, dampens the body's automatic startle response, likely due to its influence on stress regulation and nervous system modulation. You just feel more calm and less reactive after a good breathing exercise.

Years ago, we were also briefed that NASA scientists playfully tested how the WHM breathing affects the brain waves, and it seemed to show that brain waves shifted into those similar to the Dalai Lama's, which are associated with a more relaxed and focused state of mind. As we often emphasize, a relaxed body is known to facilitate increased air intake and oxygen absorption, fundamentally enhancing the depth of our breathing and opening the blood vessels. When you do the WHM breathing exercises, you can almost feel all this happening within you. All of life's worries seem to fall away, and a sense of immense trust in yourself and a clarity about the world take over. It's as though you enter a deep state of hypnosis.

Isabelle: My first experience with breathwork was at twenty-five years old. I was at home waiting to leave for a job interview, and I was very nervous and counting down the minutes! Suddenly, a conversation I'd recently had with my father popped into my head. He had told me that scientists had become curious about his breathing exercises because of how effective they seemed to be. It had been the first time his breathing techniques sparked my interest, and I had listened curiously while we were sitting in the car. So, that day, before my interview, I decided to lie down in my living room and do three rounds of around thirty breaths with exhales. I tuned in to myself more and more with every breath. I heard the ringing in my head and detached myself from my thoughts and surroundings. A sense of calm entered my body. After the exercise, I felt wowed and finally understood how amazing it was. I was energetic, clear, and calm at the same time, and my anxiousness transformed into a highly centered and motivated feeling. I was looking forward to the interview instead of feeling a sense of nervousness and resistance. Oh, and did I get the job? Yes—that, too!

The breathing acts as a full workout of the nervous and respiratory systems that profoundly changes your biochemistry—all while you're lying on a yoga mat.

Intermittent Hypoxia

During regular breathing, the body experiences only very mild fluctuation in oxygen and carbon dioxide levels. In the active breathing phase of the WHM Basic Breathing exercise, we breathe faster than we do in regular breathing, which doubles the amount of inhaled oxygen in the body and, equally important, pushes out a lot of carbon dioxide, resulting in a considerable drop in carbon dioxide concentration in the blood. During the breath holds, oxygen drops to low levels, while carbon dioxide rises.

BREAKING DOWN OXYGEN DISTRIBUTION: Inhaled oxygen is mostly distributed through our blood by red blood cells, with the help of hemoglobin, which is what the oxygen binds to on the cell. And usually, our blood oxygen saturation is already high: about 96–98 percent. During WHM breathing, blood oxygen saturation can quickly reach 100 percent.

A common question arises: How much difference can a 2–4 percent increase in oxygen saturation make to our health? While specifically looking at blood oxygen saturation, it may seem minor, but there's more to this increase. A study has shown that we double our oxygen intake during a WHM breathing practice; we simply breathe in more oxygen during the practice. During WHM breathing, the body also experiences a significant rise in oxygen dissolved directly in the plasma—oxygen that isn't bound to hemoglobin and ready to be moved to oxygen-deficient places.

It's also important to consider that oxygen doesn't just stay in the blood—it's eventually meant to go to the tissues, which always have a naturally lower oxygen concentration than the bloodstream. The oxygen transported by blood is essential for reaching individual cells, which make up tissues and organs. Our hypothesis is that this additional oxygen does much more than just elevate blood oxygen saturation by 2–4 percent. It supports improved oxygenation at the cellular level in the tissues, where it may enhance cellular detoxification, rejuvenation, and function; energy production; and tissue health. Although more research is needed looking into this matter. Then, during the retention phase, oxygen levels can temporarily drop significantly. After a minute or so in the retention, monitors show that oxygen levels start to drop. This is when we train with short moments of low oxygen levels, reaping the effects of intermittent hypoxia.

When we practice breath holds in the retention phase, our oxygen levels drop and our carbon dioxide levels rise. Interestingly, it's not actually low oxygen levels but the rise in carbon dioxide levels that triggers our breathing reflex (giving us the urge to breathe). And because we expelled a lot of carbon dioxide during the active phase, our breathing reflex kicks in later than normal, which means we can hold our breath for longer without feeling an overwhelming urge to breathe again. Even with the very first breathing session, it's not abnormal to hold your breath for as long as two minutes! When the breathing reflex finally kicks in, we take a deep breath in and hold it for around fifteen seconds. With this last big breath, you complete one full round of WHM Basic Breathing.

For a few moments toward the end of the retention phase, oxygen levels can drop significantly. In the hospital, when oxygen saturation falls below 90 percent, it signals that immediate medical attention is required. One time, Wim was doing his breathing exercises while hooked up to an oxygen saturation monitor in the hospital, and his oxygen saturation levels fell to 40 percent. The doctors rushed in but saw that Wim was doing just fine. They thought the machine was broken and replaced it with another. But when that machine also showed an impossibly low oxygen level, they understood that it was not the machine but Wim's breathing exercises. This low level of oxygen might sound alarming, but according to researchers at Radboud University Medical School, it's very unlikely to be detrimental to our cells when it's only for a few moments. Each cell has four oxygen molecules that can attach to it. When oxygen levels drop temporarily, these molecules are released one by one, and as soon as oxygen becomes available again, the cell quickly replenishes the oxygen it lost.

This phenomenon of temporarily inducing low oxygen levels in the blood and tissues is called "intermittent hypoxia." Continuous oxygen deprivation would be detrimental to the body; however, controlled intermittent hypoxia acts as a hormetic stressor and offers various benefits. In fact, many professional athletes engage in intermittent hypoxia training as part of their fitness regimen because it stimulates adaptations in the body, such as improved oxygen utilization and increased red blood cell production, which can enhance performance at sea level. This is often done by training in high-altitude locations, with simulated altitude training devices, or in low-oxygen chambers. It is also the reason why Wim could climb Mount Everest up to the death zone without any oxygen tanks.

When we enter a hypoxic state, the body reacts immediately by triggering something called hypoxia-inducible factor (HIF-1). HIF-1 plays an important role in over one hundred genes essential for survival in low levels of oxygen, like those influencing the formation of new blood vessels, the production of new red blood cells, and glycolysis—a form of energy production that doesn't rely on oxygen. Research shows that intermittent hypoxia increases levels of

LOW-OXYGEN ENVIRONMENT IN THE WOMB: Interestingly, adapting to low oxygen happens when we are embryos lying comfortably in our moms' bellies. Right at the beginning of pregnancy, when an embryo is just starting to take shape and various organs are forming and tissues are growing rapidly, HIF-1 acts as the master organizer that makes sure everything happens smoothly. Its job is to ensure that all the cells in the embryo get the oxygen and nutrients they need to thrive and grow. HIF-1 also directs the cells in their movements and helps them specialize into different types. In this sense, it's like the conductor of an orchestra.

erythropoietin (EPO), which increases the production of red blood cells and triggers the creation of new veins. As we learned before, increased numbers of red blood cells affect oxygen availability in the body because they are oxygen carriers, and veins are the roads to carry these. EPO is sometimes taken as a doping drug by athletes wanting to increase their endurance. Lance Armstrong had to hand in his seven cups because he took EPO. If only he had known about the WHM back then, he would have had a natural and legitimate way to increase his EPO production.

When we do WHM breathing, the pathways that deliver oxygen to cells react and adapt to become more fit for future oxygen shortages. The result of short-term low oxygen levels is increased lung capacity, improved circulation, cellular oxygen uptake, and improved metabolic efficiency in the long term. It also releases large amounts of adrenaline. In fact, the Radboud study found that participants practicing breathing exercises produced more adrenaline than someone bungee jumping for the first time. This creates a similar hormetic response where the body experiences a short-term spike in adrenaline, which triggers an anti-inflammatory response. As Dr. Epel explains in *The Stress Prescription*, "the higher the adrenaline spike, the better the anti-inflammatory response." All together, this creates downstream health benefits and an increased ability to handle adrenaline-charged situations in life, whether they be threatening or exciting. When you know this, you're not surprised that many people report having more energy as a result of their Wim Hof Method practice.

THE WHM VERSUS MT. KILIMANJARO: In 2014, a group of twenty-six trekkers, both men and women with limited or no prior climbing experience, accomplished a remarkable feat by not only ascending one of the world's highest mountains—Kilimanjaro, at 5,895 meters—but also reaching the summit in record time. Their achievement, which was made even more incredible by the fact that many of the trekkers suffered from medical conditions like MS, rheumatoid arthritis, and even cancer—was published through a document in a letter to the *Wilderness & Environmental Medicine* journal. Trained by Wim Hof, the group practiced the WHM to mitigate acute mountain sickness (AMS). Despite experts in mountaineering predicting it would never work—due to the rapid ascent and extreme altitude—the results were astonishing.

Typically, it takes five to seven days for trekkers to reach Kilimanjaro's summit, with a success rate of 61 percent among individuals without chronic health conditions. However, the group trained by Wim Hof accomplished the ascent within forty-eight hours, with an impressive 92 percent reaching the summit. None of the trekkers exhibited severe AMS based on standardized testing, nor did they report symptoms of hypocapnia resulting from hyperventilation, which is another common effect of the climb.

Traditionally, trekkers also use the medication Diamox to prevent high-altitude sickness, but the participants in this study did not utilize any preventive measures besides the Wim Hof Method. This expedition showcases the incredible adaptations the WHM breathing causes, and the potential of the WHM as a natural alternative for preventing severe high-altitude sickness. In one study, the efficacy of Diamox and WHM breathing was compared as antidotes against acute mountain sickness, and it showed that the WHM was just as effective.

Breathing Mechanics and Lung Capacity

When you do regular WHM breathing, you will notice your everyday breathing becomes much more optimal, and you'll benefit from a more relaxed body and mind. The specific type of deep breathing we do in the WHM engages the diaphragm, massages the organs, and strengthens the pelvic floor muscles, which creates more stability in the core and all the mechanics of the female body. Lung sacs are very elastic; when you breathe normally, their surface area stretches to around seventy square meters but can potentially expand to up to one hundred square meters. With deep breathing, the lungs expand further, and the alveoli can stretch more, increasing the available surface area for gas exchange. Over time this can lead to increased lung capacity and more efficient exchange of oxygen and carbon dioxide. And the beauty is that it doesn't take weeks or months of conscious training; it happens naturally in as little as fifteen to twenty minutes a day. In a pilot study published in 2023, researchers measured the effect of WHM breathing on the lung capacity of eleven men and women with spinal cord injuries. This condition can leave you paralyzed from the middle down and make it difficult to fully engage the lungs and diaphragm for deep breathing. Lung capacity was measured through forced vital capacity (FVC), the largest amount of air that you can forcefully exhale after breathing in as deeply as you can, and forced expiratory volume (FEV), which is the amount of air you can force from your lungs in one second. The results showed that WHM breathing led to an increase in lung capacity, measured by a significant increase in both FVC and FEV. Some participants even felt tingling sensations in parts of their bodies that were paralyzed.

Detox and Alkalization

"We are alkalizing the body" is something you'll hear Wim say time and time again in relation to WHM breathing. Although we realize this topic is a bit controversial, we deem it important to address. Our blood is slightly alkaline, with a pH of around 7.4. This is a tightly regulated process, and our internal ecosystem works best with a healthy alkalinity-to-acidity balance. Nearly every electrical and chemical event that takes place inside us—such as converting food into energy, oxidation, activation of the stress response, metabolizing and breaking down hormones, immune activation, and cleaning up environmental toxins—has an acidifying effect. With more stress and hormone-based factors, women's bodies are constantly working overtime to fight off extra acidity. The kidneys and the lungs get rid of almost all this excessive acidity; we either breathe it out via carbon dioxide, breathing faster when we need to lower acidity, or the kidneys sense our blood pH is low and filter hydrogen ions if we are too acidic, which then are excreted through the bladder. But there is a limit to the amount of toxins and acid they can process at once. If the workload is too heavy, then the substances keep circulating in the bloodstream. If systems start to fail, calcium (a powerful alkaline substance) is taken from our bones to neutralize the acids. This disruption in the acid-alkaline balance can result in an unhealthy bodily ecosystem, as it repeatedly dips into the body's alkaline reserve. When this happens in the long run, it becomes an underlying factor in a wide range of diseases.

We occasionally provide pH strips to our participants to measure their pH levels, and the results consistently show that WHM breathing can temporarily shift blood pH toward alkalinity, which may support various physiological processes. The Radboud study showed that during WHM breathing, blood pH could reach a value of 7.8, before normalizing back to 7.4 quickly after stopping the breathing.

With deep breathing, we stimulate the lymphatic system, a network of tissues, vessels, and organs that support the immune system and help the body remove waste and maintain fluid balance. We also stimulate the movement of cerebrospinal fluid (CFS), a fluid that acts as a cushion for your brain and spinal cord, nourishing them and promoting waste removal. CFS typically moves from the base of your spine to the top of your brain, using valves at both ends, about four to five times per day. However, when we do WHM breathing—the basic, but especially the power version—this fluid moves much more rapidly, clearing waste products in the brain. We potentially also increase oxygen levels in parts of the brain where inflammation has built up.

Laura: When I used to party in the good old days, I loved my red wine. But it also gave me the worst hangovers! The first time I did the breathing exercises, I was twenty-three and in need of an emergency hangover cure. I did three whole rounds of breathing together with my dad, and I looked at his face afterward with wide-open eyes and said: "Holy shit, this shit really works!" I have been hooked ever since. My headache was gone, and it felt like a dark cloud had moved out of the way. I felt lighter, and I could function again at 80 percent capacity, instead of wanting to squander the day in bed. I used the breathing exercises quite a lot during my twenties for this purpose alone.

We use the WHM breathing exercises to positively influence the nervous system as well as the respiratory system, but also some of the fundamental biochemistry of our body. We can influence anything from digestion, metabolism, and immunity to eyesight, sexual arousal, and blood pressure—all through the breath. Through manipulating the breath, you can truly become your own alchemist. And this expands not only to your body, but your mind and spirit, as well.

WHM BREATHING: FROM CLOUDS TO CLARITY

We know the nervous system affects how we breathe, with emotions like anger causing us to take quick, shallow breaths that further activate our sympathetic nervous system. We know the reverse is true: we can use the breath to settle our nervous system. With the WHM, we activate and relax at the same time. At its core, WHM breathing is about putting you in the best physical and emotional state to handle all that life throws at you, enabling you to tackle your day—with its long list of work and life tasks—with grace. After just one session of WHM breathing, the emotional charge of a stressful situation is brought back to realistic levels. The clouds of sadness, resentment, insecurity, frustration, and shame will part, and you'll feel more in balance.

Isabelle: When I have a question in life or need to make an important decision, I find that the WHM Basic Breathing exercise is an excellent way to get the right answer, as you deeply connect with your subconscious, your intuition, and your feelings. There lies a rich well of wisdom and clarity within you, and an answer will likely pop up during or after the breathing exercise!

One of the most powerful and beautiful things about women is the richness of their emotional lives, which are closely linked to the breath. The WHM breathing exercises help you connect with your heart and release emotional baggage you may be carrying around. As modern human beings, we are incredibly reliant on our prefrontal cortex, which makes up about 10 percent of our brain and is always busy analyzing and planning. Because it's working so hard, the prefrontal cortex sucks up a lot of the blood and oxygen, withholding these critical elements from other parts of your brain, where your emotions and creativity lie. When we do the breathing exercises, we disperse the blood and oxygen flow during the breath holds, letting them enter deeper regions of your brain, where your emotions are processed, and your brain stem, where your subconscious lies. This part of the brain is also where our brain and gut connect and contains an ocean full of information that we can tap into. This phenomenon was shown in the brain scan study done in Michigan in 2018. When Wim did the breathing exercises, the regions associated with self-reflection and internal focus were significantly more active, inducing a "here and now" state. This leads to less worry about the past or future by creating space in the head. These results are especially important for women, who ruminate more and who as we know have higher "fear zone" activity during stress. With the breath, we break the loop of stress in the mind, creating more space between the trigger and response.

Simultaneously, during the breath holds, where we have short moments of low oxygen levels, less blood flow goes to the prefrontal cortex, the thinking brain. This is why we can experience strong emotions while still feeling calm and safe. People with trauma often report finally being able to face their trauma and release it through WHM Power Breathing. As we enter our subconscious, we can travel along certain neurological pathways without the emotional trigger. As we explained earlier, by inducing a controlled stressor through the breath, you can confront whatever emotions while remaining calm. This creates an opportunity to reshape your relationship with past traumas that normally are strongly connected to emotions like fear and stress. This has to do with vagus nerve activity, the lowering of the pain threshold, the release of internal chemicals called endocannabinoids and opioids—among others—and lower activity in the amygdala region while in an "active" state. The shaking up of the nervous system also means that stored emotions in the body can be released and processed in a "safe" environment. One time, we led a WHM breathing exercise for a group of teenagers with behavioral issues. During the session, one of the children shared an extraordinary experience. The teenager saw his deceased mother and felt a profound connection with her, and unlike what he usually felt, he did not feel sadness. Instead, it was a rich and beautiful experience for him.

We recommend doing the WHM in the morning. In just one session, you can feel the rush of adrenaline through your system, and the blood flow will enter deeper regions of the brain, allowing you to start your day with an energetic sense of calm. This creates a different type of awareness, one where there is no space and time, where you are in full acceptance of and clarity in the present moment. An exploratory study from researchers at Washington University in St. Louis also showed that participants doing a WHM-like breathing exercise reported a heightened sense of awareness, more experiences of awe, and higher levels of perceived physical buzzing or tingling compared to the control group. It is in these moments that we learn how to use the breath as the remote control of our nervous system, steering ourselves back to calm and clarity in moments of extreme stress. We may feel an incredible connection between our body and mind, and through this connection we gain greater control over our deeper physiological processes. Sometimes, our consciousness shifts during these breath holds, as we are not breathing for minutes, and people report feeling like they don't even exist during those minutes. This is the complete stillness of the mind that the breath can give us: from clouds to clarity. Coming back, they are fully sold on the magic of the breath.

IS WHM BREATHING A PSYCHEDELIC? If you do the Wim Hof Method of breathing long enough, you will have experiences that move beyond your conscious understanding. Visualizations, past life regressions, out-of-body experiences, seeing geometric shapes, and rewatching traumatic experiences from a healthy and compassionate distance are some of the regular results of a good session. You enter a state of consciousness that's akin to what's provided by ayahuasca or powerful plant medicine. The breathwork induces changes of the balance of the body and brain's carbon dioxide and oxygen levels, which lead to shifts in consciousness.

Endogenous N,N-dimethyltryptamine (DMT) is a molecule made by the body that is only released when you are born, when you die, and during certain experiences like ayahuasca ceremonies. Despite extensive research, the source and function of endogenous DMT remain elusive. However, several theories have been proposed. One prevalent hypothesis is that the pineal gland—also known as the "seat of the soul"—serves as the body's DMT factory. Dr. Rick Strassman, a psychiatrist and author of *DMT: The Spirit Molecule: A Doctor's Revolutionary Research into the Biology of Near-Death and Mystical Experiences*, popularized the idea that the brain releases significant amounts of this compound during dreaming and at the moment of death, potentially explaining the vivid imagery experienced during sleep and near-death experiences.

Interestingly, DMT, which is also known as the spirit molecule, might be released during Wim Hof Method breathing exercises, explaining the altered states of consciousness many people experience. This still requires scientific exploration and is currently the topic of a study we are exploring with the University of Pisa.

It's clear that we get much more heart centered when we do the breathing. We experience less fear and stress, and we can act from a place of safety. When we breathe deeply, we expand the lungs and increase the blood flow in this region, which expands the heart.

WHM BREATHING PROTOCOLS

First, a word of caution: breathing exercises have a profound effect on motor control and, in rare cases, can lead to loss of consciousness. Always sit or lie down when practicing these techniques. Never practice in or near bodies of water, while driving, or in any other situation where losing consciousness could cause severe harm to you or others.

Protocol 1: The WHM Basic Breathing Exercise

The Wim Hof Method style of breathing utilizes all the things you can do with your breath: intense breathing (which is energizing), extremely long breath holds (which are relaxing), holding the breath on the exhale to create air hunger, holding the breath on the inhale after creating air hunger. These varied techniques optimize the oxygen uptake of your body.

Don't be intimidated by the breath holds; you might find it hard to believe, but many total beginners are able to do a two-minute breath hold with ease. We recommend that you do this breathing exercise on an empty stomach. Keep your focus on your breath throughout! Let the air move in and out in a cyclical way, with no beginning or end. Thoughts will come up, but welcome the thought and let it go by following the breath. If you feel a little anxious starting out, our advice is to start slow, use the nose for your inbreaths, and breathe a little deeper, slower, and exhale longer with pursed lips. You can slowly build up the tempo.

1. GET COMFORTABLE: Close your eyes and clear your mind. Shift your attention to your heart. Start tuning in to your breathing, fully connecting with each breath. Focus on inhaling deeply and actively through your nose or mouth, and then release an unforced exhale through your mouth in short, powerful bursts. Breathe fully into your belly, then your chest, and release the air naturally without forcing it. Repeat this process thirty to forty times and make it circular. During this, you may experience lightheadedness or tingling sensations in your body.

2. BREATH HOLD: After completing the thirty to forty deep breaths, take one deeper inhale, filling your lungs to their maximum capacity without straining. Then exhale and hold your breath for as long as you comfortably can.

3. RECOVERY BREATH: When you feel the need to breathe again, take one deep breath in, expanding your belly and chest fully. Hold this breath for ten to fifteen seconds, then release. This completes one round of the exercise. You can repeat this breathing exercise for three to four rounds consecutively.

After you have completed the breathing exercise, take your time and enjoy the feeling. We recommend relaxing completely for five to fifteen minutes in meditation. This is the moment we can gain deep insights. I (Laura) often end my breathing with a "plant a seed" meditation when I am teaching. I ask people to come up with a heartfelt goal or wish and plant it in their subconscious so they can manifest it in their reality. I often have people contact me after my retreats, telling me how powerful this exercise has been in manifesting their dreams.

Protocol 2: On-the-Go Stress Relief

Sometimes when we're running around, sleeping poorly, and rushing from task to task all day, it causes us to fall into an unhealthy breathing pattern of taking shallow breaths into the chest. This can leave us feeling stressed and tired, with a lot of pressure and tightness in the chest. If you find yourself in this situation, take a moment to pause and do the following exercise.

1. Feel what you are experiencing. What do you feel in your body? And where are you feeling it?
2. Accept the feeling and give yourself a pat on the shoulder to acknowledge that you are aware of this moment and feeling.
3. The breath is at this moment the most important thing in your life, so let's deepen it. Connect with the breath. Take a deep breath into your belly, expanding the abdominal area and whole rib cage. Do this as slowly as possible.
4. Breathe out deeply and try to expand the exhale, making whatever sound you want, if that feels right.
5. Stop for a moment after breathing out.
6. Repeat this ten times—or more, if you wish. Feel yourself soften and the energy returning into your body with every breath.

Isabelle: When I feel tired or stressed, and don't have the time to do the WHM breathing exercise, I engage in this mindful breathing exercise, and by focusing on my breath and body, I feel my energy is replenished.

Protocol 3: Reduce Pelvic Floor Pain

Developed by Wim, this protocol is specifically designed to target the pelvic floor to reduce symptoms or any type of pelvic floor dysfunction.

1. Stand comfortably and close your eyes, shifting your focus from what's outside to what's going on within you.

2. Take ten deep and conscious breaths, in and out, with intent. Make sure your breaths are as full and deep as they can be. Use your nose or mouth, whatever makes you take in the air better, and mouth for the exhale.

3. On the tenth breath, breathe in fully and close your mouth.

4. Now, slowly bend at the hips, moving your torso all the way down, as far as you can go naturally without force, and "hang." Press the air into your pelvic floor as if you were trying to go to the bathroom. Wiggle your hips a bit, keeping them loose.

5. Allow your attention to go to any stress you may be feeling and, as we say, "bless the stress" and try to let it release.

6. After ten to fifteen seconds of holding your breath, slowly release while still bending forward.

7. Slowly move back up to a standing position.

8. Repeat however many times you'd like.

Protocol 4: Power Breathing (DMT)

This Power Breathing, which we also call DMT breathing, can be intense, but it is an amazing method of trauma release. It will propel you to extraordinary states of consciousness, allowing you to delve deeper into the realms of your mind and making for a profound and transformative journey. This method is more intense than the WHM Basic Breathing exercise, leading to more powerful results. Practitioners may encounter intense and uncontrollable emotions, along with physical sensations such as chills along the spine and waves of electrical energy coursing through the body. Due to its intensity, we recommend only doing the Power Breathing exercise when you are well-versed in the WHM Basic Breathing exercise or, even better, when under the supervision of a WHM instructor. For one round of WHM Power Breathing, repeat the following steps:

1. Relax: Sit or lie down.
2. Complete sixty deep breaths, inhaling fully and letting your breath go. Maintain the normal WHM breathing rhythm while starting (first gear). Fasten the rhythm after twenty breaths (second gear), and again after the following twenty breaths (third gear).
3. After sixty breaths, take a full inhale.
4. Exhale the last breath fully.
5. Inhale deeply once more.
6. Hold your breath for ten to fifteen seconds, squeezing your entire body and creating slight pressure toward your head.
7. Let your breath go and move to the next round.

A full exercise of WHM Power Breathing is three to six rounds.

Protocol 5: Breathe Like a Monk

Six breaths per minute is considered ideal for everyday breathing, and interestingly, this is also the breathing pace that monks naturally assume during meditation without any formal training. This type of breathing grounds you in the present moment and allows you to observe your emotional state and self-regulate.

1. Find a comfortable seat and relax your body, releasing any tension. Focus on your breath.
2. Use a clock to time each breath, inhaling and exhaling for ten seconds each. Imagine you are breathing from the heart, allowing the air to fill your belly.
3. As you settle into the rhythm, you may feel "in the zone." At this point, close your eyes, maintain the pace, and count silently without looking at the clock.
4. Once you feel comfortable maintaining the pace naturally, stop counting and let your body regulate the timing without conscious effort.

5. Stay in this calm state for a few minutes, or as long as you like. You'll experience a sense of calm and presence, fully anchored in the moment.

To establish the habit, practice this breathing exercise daily. Enjoy the peace and Zen-like satisfaction of breathing like a monk.

After years of teaching WHM breathing, we have seen thousands of women use these exercises to deal with their trauma, boost their energy levels, and finally bring their nervous system into a state of peace and calm. In the following chapter, we'll learn how to combine the power of the breath and the cold to create life-changing mindset shifts.

MINDSET:
FROM WORRIER TO WARRIOR

"Relax, nothing is under control."

A few years ago, a woman attended one of our workshops. Like many other women who come to our trainings, she walked in tentatively and was a little shy at first. She was most hesitant about the ice bath, and admitted she was terrified to enter the cold, especially in front of a bunch of people she'd just met. And although she had a hard time getting in and staying in at first, by the end of the day, she had successfully completed her first ice bath.

Talking to her at the end of the training was like talking to a different person. The courageous act of getting into the cold and trying something outside her comfort zone gave her an immediate newfound confidence. She had certainly conquered a personal challenge at the workshop, but at the time, we didn't realize the massive impact it would have on her outside the training. Her mindset had undergone a significant shift, and she began trusting herself in ways she never had before. A while after the workshop, she reached out to let us know that she had done something she'd wanted to do for years—quit her job and started her own company. The WHM sparked a massive neurological redirection, shifting her mindset from "I can't" to "I can." It gave her the courage to make a scary decision that changed the course of her life.

The transformations we see in the women who attend our trainings are truly mind-blowing. So many women walk into our workshops and retreats brimming with anxiety and self-consciousness, but leave—after just a few hours—suddenly oozing a calm, contagious confidence. The method is an extremely effective way to silence the fearful, anxious saboteur in our own head and ignite the determined, fearless warrior we all carry within. After all, the biggest challenge women face when coming to the workshop isn't really the ice bath—it's what it represents in our life: a goal, an obstacle, a limiting belief, past trauma, or our deepest fears or insecurities. Conquering the ice bath means conquering your comfort zone and entering your personal growth zone.

When we talk about shifting mindset, it doesn't only mean making it work more efficiently. As we already know from Chapter 2, most women have extremely active minds and are already able to trigger multiple parts of the brain simultaneously, firing off more neuronal activity than men. Instead, it's about slowing down and connecting the body and the mind, learning to harness the incredible power of the mind-body connection. By tapping into this incredible connection, we become conscious masters of our own destiny.

THE SCIENCE OF THE MIND-BODY (DIS)CONNECTION

The science of the connection between the mind and the body has been the source of much discussion and debate. For centuries, in many major cultures and religions, the mind and body were seen as inseparable. René Descartes, a sixteenth-century mathematician and scientific thinker, was one of the first to challenge this belief, arguing that the mind and the body are entirely separate entities. His theory played a significant role in shaping Western beliefs about the mind-body connection, setting the groundwork for many modern medical breakthroughs but also contributing to Western medicine's ignorance of how the mind affects the body. This has led to significant gaps in treatment, as the mind-body connection can have a massive influence on not just the development of disease but also the treatment of it. While the field of neuroscience is still uncovering the science of the mind-body connection, there are countless examples of how the mind influences the body, and the body influences the mind. And we cannot fully understand either when we see them as separate entities.

THE HOMUNCULUS AND THE (HER)MUNCULUS: In 1936, the neurosurgeon Wildon Penfield created a visual representation of the connections between parts of the body and parts of the brain. It was called the cortical homunculus (Latin for "little man"), and it became a key resource in medical and neuroscience textbooks. The representation—although very distorted—shows where the motor and sensory functions in the brain are in relation to the body. By stimulating a specific brain region in the representation, one could trace the resulting sensation to the corresponding area of the body. This vividly demonstrated the existence of a mind-body connection, illustrating their inseparability. That said, historically only about 0.5 to 1 percent of brain research is performed on women, so female brains were more or less not accounted for in the cortical homunculus. Recently, an effort has been made to also create a representation of the female brain, which has been named the "hermunculus."

Communication between the brain and body happens through incredibly fast and powerful chemical and electrical signals. Think about this: we only need to visualize biting into a lemon to experience the effect of increased saliva in our mouth. Similarly, the best athletes in the world use visualization techniques to get ahead of the game by improving motor skills and even growing muscle strength. We know that playing the piano in your head can make you a better pianist, and watching tennis can improve your game on the actual court. The act of mental rehearsal, or visualization, is so potent because our subconscious mind processes the experience as a real one and fires the same neurological pathways that are responsible for the acquired skill.

Placebo and Nocebo

Other concrete examples of how our mind can influence our physical reality are the placebo and nocebo effects, which describe a scientifically proven phenomenon where a patient's perception of a treatment can actually influence its success or failure. In one study, Harvard professor Dr. Alia Crum measured the impact of mindset on the physical health markers of eighty-four women working in hotel housekeeping. She divided the participants into two groups: one was told that the amount of physical activity they did while working met the criteria for an "active lifestyle," and the second didn't receive this information. Although both groups of ladies did the same amount of work and exercise, group one—the informed "placebo" group— thought they had been much more active when they received the same question after four weeks. And it wasn't only their perception that changed; so did their real-life results. On average the women in group one lost two pounds, compared to the control group, who didn't lose any weight, and their blood pressure decreased significantly as well. The effects were carefully monitored, and the results were adjusted for food intake and any other exercise the women had done. The researchers concluded that mindset and belief significantly affected the physical health of this group of women. In another example, studies have shown that sugar pills can be just as effective at relieving pain as morphine. It's clear through research using brain scans that positive expectation or belief can influence real-life results.

The opposite, the nocebo effect, is also true. If you expect a medicine or treatment will not work or that it will give you negative side effects, your body and mind will conspire to make you correct! In one study, people given fake poison actually developed rashes when exposed to a completely benign substance.

Clearly, thoughts and beliefs have a tangible effect on our physiology. Every thought we have activates specific neurological pathways that are linked to bodily functions via the nervous system. Every thought in your head leaves a physical trace or footprint, just like a well-traveled path in a forest. When you think certain thoughts often or long enough, this path gets stronger, wider, deeper, and more ingrained. Allow it to be present long enough, and the thought becomes a belief that starts to define your actions and physical reality, stored in your brain. This isn't just mental; it's physically happening in your brain and body.

Signs of a Mind-Body Disconnection

What's most surprising about the effect of this powerful connection is that so few people are aware of it and how it might be sabotaging their health. There are so many aspects of our modern lifestyle (think: social media, a sedentary lifestyle, lack of connection with others) that put us at risk for a disconnected mind and body. This is true especially for women, whose minds are incredibly active. In the female brain, the prefrontal cortex—the part of the brain involved in worrying and analyzing—uses up a lot of the brain's resources thinking about yesterday or tomorrow instead of being in the here and now. As we learned in Chapter 2, women naturally have more connectivity to and within the amygdala, also known as the "fear center" of our brain. Women also have more connectivity and activity within and to the default mode network (DMN) parts of the brain, which play a role in rumination and worries, and are pretty much in the background constantly assessing every situation, asking: Am I safe? This is an evolutionary adaptation that is supposed to help us out, but these days, our fight-or-flight response is triggered by thoughts and an overactive brain that is in a state of high vigilance, which can invoke an intense reaction in our bodies and interfere with our mind-body connection. Our minds are constantly being triggered; we are programmed to react quicker to negative stimuli than positive, and we are extremely good at thinking in endless loops! The consequence of all this is that we are fully "in our heads" instead of connected with our bodies.

So how do you know if you are struggling with an overactive mind, and a disconnected mind-body connection? Here are some telltale signs:

- Suppressing, ignoring, and avoiding your emotions
- Substance abuse
- Overeating
- Avoiding difficult situations
- Not being in tune with your intuition or heart
- Poor emotional regulation
- Feeling overwhelmed by emotions
- Having a tendency toward overthinking or indecision
- Feeling disconnected from the body
- Being overly reliant on the mind
- Always overstepping your physical boundaries until it's too late
- Not being able to catch subtle cues from your body

Gabor Maté, a Canadian physician and the author of many leading books on psychology and mindset, described the profound effect the mind-body connection plays in the development of disease in women. He explains that women's tendency to not be able to say no, be overly caring, sacrifice themselves, not have enough self-respect, be too complacent, and repress their own needs and emotions sets them up for harm in the long term. Because while the mind may be able to keep pushing, the body, as Maté explains, will eventually be the one to say no, and usually this is in the form of illness. In Maté's book *When the Body Says No*, he explains that emotional stress is often a major contributor to breast cancer, as research shows that major stress moments have often precipitated the onset of the disease. This may also contribute to the reality that women are twice as likely to suffer from severe stress, anxiety, and depression as men.

It's not just the biological differences between men and women that affect the mind-body connection; women also face the massive challenge of society's expectations on them, which have weighed heavy on women's psyches for centuries.

FEMALE CONDITIONING

A woman's sense of self is not shaped by neurology alone; it's formed by a variety of genetic, biological, social, economic, and cultural factors. From a social and cultural perspective, women have been raised and conditioned to act according to certain expectations that are often stricter for them than those that men face. And although there have been several steps taken toward the emancipation of women from these stereotypes in the past decades, we think we can all agree it is still a man's world.

Even modern society teaches women that we should listen instead of talk, that we cannot decide for ourselves, and that we need a man and children to be considered successful. This "Barbie syndrome," as we like to call it, teaches us to be pretty, sweet, submissive, and agreeable, and to put ourselves in second place behind our fathers, husbands, children, and brothers. All around the world, women receive the message, either subtly and subconsciously or very clearly and consciously, that we are only lovable if we can fulfill the many, many expectations society has of us. America Ferrera's character in the *Barbie* movie summed it up well when she said:

> It is literally impossible to be a woman. . . . Like, we have to always be extraordinary, but somehow we're always doing it wrong.
>
> You have to be thin, but not too thin. . . . You have to be a boss, but you can't be mean. You have to lead, but you can't squash other people's ideas. You're supposed to love being a mother, but don't talk about your kids all the damn time. . . .
>
> It's too hard! It's too contradictory and nobody gives you a medal or says thank you! And it turns out in fact that not only are you doing everything wrong, but also everything is your fault.

Overcoming this Barbie syndrome is much bigger than just trying to make different decisions. For us to break free, we need to tap into our own deepest desires and needs. Only then can we truly embrace our individuality and trust ourselves to confidently forge our own way in life—regardless of what society thinks.

BREAKING THROUGH CONDITIONING

We have seen time and time again that the Wim Hof Method helps women reclaim their power in the face of self-doubt and societal expectations. The breathing exercises enable us to observe our thoughts from a healthy distance, instead of being consumed by them or reacting immediately. The ice bath trains us to be less reactive and fearful, to stay in and face the cold instead of doing the easiest thing and immediately jumping out. When we can observe our conditioned behavior and override this instinct during the ice bath, it teaches us what we're capable of, inside and outside the ice, in our everyday lives.

It also allows us to create more awareness of our thoughts and beliefs, and not attach so much meaning to them. We can ask ourselves follow-up questions about the thoughts in our head, such as: Is this

---

Laura: I had a mantra when I was six years old. For a whole year I would tell everybody (dancing while I said it): "I can do whatever I want." What an empowering message! Being able to do and be whatever I want? I rehearsed this sentence with a full-on attitude and movement, and the saying—as well as the intention and deeper meaning behind it—became encoded into my nervous system and subconscious mind. I have traveled the world alone, feeling fearless, confident, safe, and happy! I have been happy to go against the grain many times, speaking up in meetings without hesitation, and have often chosen a less popular path that felt aligned with my own happiness even though the whole world seemed to go the opposite way. I have never had a problem stating my opinion and am fine with people disagreeing with me. I have been taught to follow my own intuition, and that I play the main role in my life and have a different path from any other being on the planet. I always give this advice to others: follow your intuition, the quiet voice within you that is not afraid of anything. Figure out: What is it that you want? And just go get it! This is your life, not anybody else's. I believe that we become unhappy when we do not follow our own deeper inner voice; this leads to a feeling of misalignment. This is the female intuition, a greater knowing, that goes beyond the conscious mind.

thought true? Could it actually be false? How could I think or act differently? Is this thought opening me up to more possibilities, or limiting me? Far too often, our thoughts and inner voice are keeping us safe in our comfort zone. They become nervous chatter when we are confronted with challenges, keeping us away from potential growth. They say: "you can't do that," "you're not good enough," "just play it safe," or "just do what you were told." By bringing this inner voice out in a controlled setting, which is what we do when we go into an ice bath, we become aware of it and can face it head-on. The cold acts as a mirror. With the WHM, we create space in the mind for each of us to find alignment between our mind and body to strengthen our true essence. Only then can we confidently take actions that align with our deepest needs.

WHM MINDSET: MINDFULNESS 2.0

As we have learned, our minds can be our most powerful resource, but they can also be our worst enemy. When our mind is cluttered by stress, destructive thoughts, and external expectations, it will impact us physically and lead us down the wrong path. But when we feel safe and secure in our body, we can also think clearly, trust our gut to make decisions, and create the life we want.

The first step toward nurturing this mind-body connection is slowing down.

Still the Mind

Did you know studies show most adults spend half their time wondering about the past and/or future? The Dutch have a saying: "The one who stands with one leg in the past and one in the future pisses over the present." While this phrase is really only catchy in Dutch, the meaning behind the words is clear even in English. The foundation of the WHM mindset pillar is stilling the mind to bring yourself in the here and now, so you can make the best of the present moment.

The WHM is a powerful tool for this, far more effective for many people than other mindfulness techniques, like yoga or meditation. We have had many people share that they were not able to meditate before finding the Wim Hof Method, but as soon as they discovered the breathing exercises, they could calm their mind easily. This makes perfect sense to us. Tell a stressed, busy woman to sit down and meditate. Their minds go crazy! The WHM uses the power of breathwork and cold exposure to create an experience akin to mindfulness 2.0. When we go into an ice bath, the blood is directed to the most primal part of the brain, which means the prefrontal cortex is less active and we experience fewer racing thoughts and future worries, a less active "monkey mind." Go sit in an ice bath and think about your troubles. You can't! You can only *be*. There is no space for the past or future, only the present moment. One of the big benefits of quieting our mind is that it allows us to connect more with our body and pay attention to what it's telling us. Research into the WHM, still to be published, showed that the WHM is also superior to meditation.

Foster Interoception

After we slow down and still the mind, we can start to pay attention to what's going on internally. In our trainings, we often refer to this as your inner world, which includes factors like heart rate, breathing, temperature, hunger, energy level, and pain but also any emotions like sadness, anger, or joy hanging out underneath the surface. Change always starts with awareness; by getting more in tune with your body, you take the first step toward regulating your physiology and emotions. Studies show that the insula, the part of the brain responsible for self-reflection that is strengthened through meditation, also increases with Wim Hof Method practice. You can only change and regulate when you are aware of something. This works in strange and beautiful ways. When we get into the cold, there's an immediate, short-term drop of activity in the insula, but a longer-term increase after the practice. We rewire our brain and expand our consciousness.

Interoception plays a pivotal role in our lives. For example, when your body doesn't feel safe, it will lead to a slight increase in tension in the chest or a slightly elevated heartbeat. If you're able to notice this right away, you can take steps to either reassure your body that it's safe or to remedy the situation, instead of allowing your anxiety and fear to build up, possibly turning into something more extreme, like a panic attack.

The WHM has been shown to increase our interoceptive focus abilities, as measured in brain scans. Practicing the method led to activation in regions of the brain associated with self-reflection and control, as well as a part in the brainstem that can "soothe" and have an analgesic effect. In another study into the WHM, subjects reported a greater connection to their thoughts and feelings. Research shows that the heart and gut have more nerves going to the brain than the other way around, proving that it is part of our fundamental human design to listen to our body and our gut. Through much of human history, our survival depended on our ability to listen to the intelligence of our bodies.

The ability to have an internal set of ears always listening to the subtle cues of the body is invaluable for anyone, but especially for women since our physiology can change greatly throughout our monthly cycles and our lives, with pregnancy and menopause. Interoceptive focus helps us understand our changing internal states during these transitions and adjust our needs. Research shows that a woman's brain changes dramatically during the menstrual cycle (many of us can relate to the term "emotional roller coaster"). The mind-body connection we foster with the WHM can help us tap into the intelligence of bodies during our cycle to maintain a better sense of control and balance.

VISUALIZATION OF SUCCESS: Visualization is simply a mental rehearsal. We create images in our mind of having or doing whatever it is we want. Visualization works directly on the brain, altering brain-wave activity and biochemistry; in fact, scientific studies have shown the positive effects of creative visualization on health, including immunity, stress, healing, and pain management. Science also shows that it improves many facets of life, from athletic ability to cognitive performance, self-esteem, and goal achievement.

Why is it so effective? Because the brain doesn't distinguish between an action itself and thoughts about an action, so mental practices also have a physical imprint, though it is less powerful, and doing both is more effective than either one on its own. Before entering a cold source, we use visualization to program our body and mind for what is going to happen to prepare it, so it knows what to do. We visualize how it would feel to succeed and what sensations we are going to experience in the cold. But most importantly, we imagine how it will be to get out of the ice and how we are going to recover. When in the cold, visualization is also used to warm up. We can visualize a heat source such as flames or a stove in our belly or visualize ourselves in a hot environment, such as a sauna or Jacuzzi, or walking in bright sunlight. This is even more powerful when we engage all the senses in the visualization—we feel it, see it, sense it, smell it, and hear it.

Acceptance and Mental Fitness

One of the great lessons the WHM teaches us is that we might have limited control over our circumstances, but we do have control over how we respond. As we like to say in our trainings: life is full of metaphorical "ice baths." Everybody experiences difficulties, hardship, and trauma. Challenging circumstances will always exist; we can't control that. What we can control is how we deal with these challenges when they inevitably come our way. Ask yourself: When challenges arise, do you:

- Get stuck or bogged down by your emotions?
- Ignore your emotions?
- Try to control the situation?
- Push through it no matter what?
- Become scared or anxious?
- Flee or avoid the situation?
- Face your challenges head-on and allow yourself to go through a range of emotions?

The answers to these questions show what your conditioned response is toward any difficult situation in life. In the ice bath, your conditioned response to stress, to fears, to challenges will instantly come up. The physical ice bath is therefore also a metaphor for any difficult thing, limiting belief, or fear you must face in your life. Learn to deal with an ice bath, and you learn to deal with any stress you have in your life.

Because of this instinctual reaction to stress, the ice bath provides us with the opportunity to train our mind. As research into the WHM states, the individual needs an external stimulus (in this case an ice bath) to optimally concentrate or meditate. Mentally, you are either in and completely immersed in the ice bath, focused and connected with the body, or you are out—there is no in-between. There is no cheating with an ice bath, so the neural connection will be formed or strengthened right in the moment.

When we carry ourselves confidently and compassionately through an ice bath, we increase our resilience toward all "ice baths" in life. This is called cross-adaptation, which describes a phenomenon where an adaptation to one stressor can be applied to others. In one study, the WHM raised the participants' stress threshold, and seemed to work as a buffer for other types of future stressors. This means that by practicing the WHM, we are optimizing our mind-body connection so that stress influences us less quickly and intensely. In one study, researchers compared a group that practices "awareness of thoughts and feelings" with a group that practices the same thing in addition to practicing explicit acceptance of one's state, especially the negative experiences we typically push away. Both groups seemed to gain attentional benefits from the practices, but only the "acceptance" group showed an improved stress reactivity profile, indicating that acceptance leads to greater stress resilience. That is why when we teach the WHM, we focus on not just embracing the cold but also accepting it.

With the WHM, we learn to be comfortable in the uncomfortable, turning on the cold tap with a can-do attitude, and as we say to our students while they're in the ice bath: "embrace the suck" or "embrace the cold like a warm friend." This acceptance of short bouts of controlled stressful stimuli changes our physiology and ultimately leads to increased stress resilience. Acceptance is the true key to resilience.

Empowerment

The more you do the hard things in life, the more confident you become. And getting in (and staying in!) an ice bath is extremely hard. When we go into the ice bath with the right mindset and regulate ourselves in the face of extreme stress, we emerge feeling like we can do anything, benefiting from a surge of dopamine, adrenaline, and testosterone that can make us feel incredibly powerful. The exercise of the ice bath shows us that we can conquer our own mind. We regain our power and create a strong neurological connection between mind and body. When we do it, we feel incredible, like we are bursting through a ceiling we didn't even know was there. And luckily, the more we do it, the easier and more natural it becomes.

A few years ago, one of the WHM instructors—who is an inarguably intelligent and competent woman—was asked to do the science talk at one of our big events. To our surprise, she hesitated and fell into a mindset of self-doubt and fear. But, remembering her many experiences of calmly stepping into an ice bath, she reminded herself of her capability to conquer challenging tasks and found the confidence to give the presentation in front of a very large crowd. In no surprise to any of us, she was amazing! We always believed in her, but even the most competent people have self-doubts, especially women. It's up to us to prevent these false thoughts from holding us back and keeping us from growing.

Like this instructor, many women have found the ice bath to be a huge stepping stone for confidence that helped them do more things they were initially afraid of. Many people assume that confidence is something you are either born with or not, but the truth is that it is built. You build confidence by being afraid of something and doing it anyway.

WHM MINDSET PROTOCOLS

As you experiment with the Wim Hof Method and complete the 30-Day Icewoman Challenge, don't leave out the mindset exercises! These exercises might seem less tangible or challenging than the breath or mindset, but they are equally important, if not more important.

Protocol 1: Setting an Intention

This practice aligns the mind and body so you can go out and accomplish your goals. It starts with focusing on the breath and stilling the mind and then prompts you to tune in to your body and set an intention.

1. To begin, find a quiet, comfortable place to sit, and focus on following your breath.
2. Breathe in deeply, then let it go.
3. Follow the breath peacefully as you continue breathing.
4. As you follow the breath, a sense of calm will begin to settle over you.
5. Scan your body, taking your time and asking it how it feels. Be aware of any sensations you feel and just acknowledge them.
6. Once you've scanned your body and you're settled further into a place of calm, visualize what it is you are going to do. Then set an intention for your practice, to strengthen your resolve. View the challenge as that which you want to achieve or overcome. Perhaps you want to stay a little longer in the cold shower or achieve a new personal record for push-ups. Maybe you want to hold a particularly challenging yoga pose or take a longer bike ride than you ever have before.
7. You'll be able to detect any misalignment in your intention and how your body feels. If you sense this, just remain calm, keep breathing, and wait for the moment in which there is a sense of trust and alignment. Give power to that feeling.
8. Now, go and do what you intend to do. Good luck!

Protocol 2: Interoception of the Heartbeat

Many women struggle with an overactive mind, with female brains having the ability to trigger multiple parts simultaneously and fire more neuronal activity with the same thoughts than men. This practice helps you get out of your head and back into your body.

1. Sit or lie down in a safe, comfortable space.
2. Take a moment to relax.
3. Put one hand over your heart and feel and visualize your heartbeat.
4. Connect with your heartbeat and try to synchronize it with your breath.
5. Think about something you're grateful for. This can be anything, from the beautiful morning sun, to the fact that you started your day hugging your loved one, to the smell of a flower. Choose something that resonates with you.
6. Reconnect with your heartbeat and try to synchronize your breath and heartbeat again.
7. Scan through your body and try to feel your heartbeat in different parts of it. If you focus on your hand, feel the heartbeat in your little pinky, and if you focus on your feet, feel the blood flow from your ankles to your toes.

A couple of minutes per day is enough to help you deepen this connection and reap the benefits.

Understanding the three principles of the Wim Hof Method is one thing, but you're probably also wondering: What benefits will you get from doing the method? We've already touched on some of the benefits for stress, inflammation, and hormone balance—which are key to overall health and wellness—but what about specific life stages, conditions, illnesses, symptoms, and issues? That's what we'll dive into in the following chapters.

THE WHM FOR PREGNANCY, POSTPARTUM, AND MENOPAUSE

The WHM has a long list of benefits for women, but one place it really shines is easing the hormonal transitions many women experience throughout their lives. Our innate design as women to carry babies means we experience intense hormonal shifts during our lifetime. We transform from a girl to a woman who menstruates and is able to get pregnant. We may experience the incredible physiological changes of pregnancy, breastfeeding, and the postpartum period. When we say goodbye to our last egg around age fifty, we enter menopause and experience yet another shift.

These hormonal transitions accompany some of the richest and most meaningful moments of our lives. But that doesn't mean they're easy on our bodies or minds. These stages of life test our physical and emotional endurance in big ways, and we face them with remarkable strength and grace, even though we often lack support.

With the WHM, we can support our health and well-being during these delicate transitions, despite the many fluctuations and twists and turns. In this chapter, we'll review the benefits of the WHM for pregnancy, postpartum, and menopause, as well as how to adapt your practice during these times of great change.

FERTILITY AND PREGNANCY

More than any other time in history, women are waiting longer to have children. In the Netherlands, women are on average thirty years old when they have their first child, compared to twenty-nine in 2010, twenty-seven in 1990, and twenty-four in 1970. The availability of contraception, increasing career aspirations among women, and the shift in gender roles have changed family dynamics significantly in just a single generation. There are many positive things about waiting longer to have children, but the decrease in both male and female fertility with age has also led to more people struggling to get pregnant. This can be an incredibly difficult experience, one that often creates a disconnect between our mind and body.

Research shows that there's a clear link between stress and infertility, showing correlation between infertility and morning cortisol levels. Additionally, inflammation, especially in the uterus, can make it more difficult for the egg to nestle, again reducing the chance of pregnancy. It's important to work directly with a doctor if you are dealing with infertility, and we dive into PCOS and endometriosis in the next chapter, when we discuss chronic inflammatory and autoimmune diseases.

If you are trying to get pregnant, you can use the WHM to decrease stress, regulate your emotions, and fend off inflammation. We recommend practicing:

- the breathing exercises daily,
- one to two ice baths or cold dips per week for a maximum of three minutes, with gradual buildup, and
- daily cold showers (two minutes maximum) after your hot shower.

If you start creating a resilient body and mind before getting pregnant, it will give you a leg up for pregnancy but also a good kick-start in life for your baby. That said, always listen to your body, and if you feel like it's ever too much, skip a day. A positive mindset can also help reduce rumination you may be experiencing about getting pregnant, which can help you accept the situation as it is, and let go of the expectation of getting pregnant. The more regularly you use the WHM practices, the more you will support the careful design of your reproductive system.

PREGNANCY

After conception, the egg and sperm undergo a miraculous transition into a miniature human being. The hope is that when you are pregnant, you feel good both physically and emotionally, and can experience the process in all its richness. Unfortunately, this isn't always the case, as our bodies are working full-time—or really, double time!—leading to fatigue, nausea, mood changes, and other symptoms. The good news is that working with the cold, breath, and mindset can improve many of these symptoms by regulating your internal state and enhancing your physical and mental health.

As a general guideline, we advise temporarily stopping more extreme cold exposure practices like ice baths and cold water swimming in the first trimester because pregnancy can be fragile in the first three months. Instead, you can do a cold rinse at the end of your warm showers. What is most important is to connect deeply with

IS COLD/HEAT EXPOSURE SAFE WHILE PREGNANT? As female guides of the WHM, we have been asked this question many, many times. Very little research has been done on cold exposure while pregnant, but one review showed that cold exposure "poses minimal risk to the fetus." When practiced responsibly and wisely, it is considered safe. During pregnancy, you experience increased heart rate and a lower blood pressure during the first and second trimester, and cold water may further increase the heart rate and slightly increase blood pressure. As we've learned, though, the core body temperature stays warm even during cold exposure, so it's unlikely that cold exposure would affect the placental blood flow. Similarly, short sauna sessions can be a relaxing practice during pregnancy. Research shows that a core body temperature above 102.2 degrees can impose risk for the fetus, but it is extremely unlikely a sauna would raise the core body temperature above that. A systematic review regarding heat exposure mentioned that saunas up to twenty minutes at 158 degrees are safe during pregnancy, and none of the women analyzed exceeded a core body temperature of 102.2 degrees. *A note of caution: The exception to this rule is women with high-risk pregnancies. If you're unsure whether you fall into this category, you should consult your doctor or midwife before cold or heat exposure, especially if you have any cardiovascular issues.*

your intuition and to trust your body. If you are an experienced practitioner and you are feeling healthy, cold exposure in the form of ice baths in your second and third trimesters can be done occasionally in a range that feels comfortable to you. The most important thing is to not overdo it! Leave any rigid to-do lists regarding cold exposure behind; instead, go with the feeling and go with the flow.

Isabelle: When I found out I was pregnant, I stopped doing ice baths for the first trimester. When I started again, I didn't stop until one week before delivery. And I felt great doing it! However, I never overdid it. During my pregnancy, I also discussed heat exposure with my midwife, and she said it would not raise an issue for the fetus, as it was very unlikely to become overheated. I practiced my sauna visits on the lower benches and never for more than ten minutes at a time. It felt comfortable, safe, and above all, wonderful!

During the rest of pregnancy, cold exposure can be an energizing and mood-enhancing practice. One study on nonpregnant women showed that those who regularly practice cold exposure experience better moods, have less stress, feel more energetic, and benefit from a stronger immune system, which could greatly benefit women during pregnancy. Research shows that women who regularly practice cold water swimming experience improved birth outcomes, with the authors hypothesizing that the cold practice improves pain tolerance and adaptability to stress.

During pregnancy, the hormone HPL (human placental lactogen) is released to ensure there is a consistent supply of glucose for the baby. HPL does this by making glucose receptors less sensitive, which means that during pregnancy, women become 50 to 60 percent less insulin-sensitive, leaving women at risk for gestational diabetes. Research shows that cold exposure can increase insulin sensitivity, which means that cold exposure during pregnancy may guard against gestational diabetes.

The majority of women experience shortness of breath during pregnancy due to the diaphragm moving into a higher position to make space for the growing baby and uterus. Your breathing rate increases because your lung volume decreases and there is a significantly higher metabolic demand. The increase in progesterone during pregnancy contributes to this, as progesterone is a breathing stimulant.

During pregnancy, focusing on deepening the breath is very beneficial, though we don't recommend doing the WHM Basic Breathing exercise because of the breath holds and short-term moments of oxygen deprivation. Instead, we recommend the breathing practice below, which can help you breathe in a rhythmic way to regulate your nervous system and emotions. Use this practice to become mindful of the breath and body, slowly letting the air flow more easily and releasing tension in the muscles. With this practice you will enter a state of heightened awareness, and it can be a beautiful moment to connect deeply with your little one.

WHM Pregnancy Interoceptive Breathing Practice

Take a moment to pause and follow these steps:

1. Ask yourself: What do you feel in your body? How is your breath? Is it shallow or deep, slow or quick? Are you naturally breathing through your nose or your mouth?
2. Lean into your breath and deepen it.
3. Take a deep breath in through your nose, expanding your belly and then slowly expanding the whole rib cage.
4. Breathe deeply out through the mouth and try to make the exhale as long as possible.
5. Find a rhythm for your inhale and exhale and continue for a few minutes, or as long as it takes to feel your body starting to relax.
6. When you are in a state of relaxation and fully engaged with the breath, you can turn your attention to your belly. Put your hands on it and feel what is going on.
7. Envision the smile of your growing baby inside. See it, feel it, hear it. That's him/her, that is you, that is connection.

While it's important to adapt your WHM practice in pregnancy, it can be a safe and effective way to stay energized and healthy and to connect deeply with your baby.

POSTPARTUM

Congratulations, your baby is out in the world! The postpartum period is a very rich moment, as you have just added a new member to the family. At the same time, it's a very intense phase where you experience drastic physical and emotional changes. It's incredible how much attention goes into pregnancy and preparing for birth, and how little to postpartum.

During this time your hormone constitution is shifting yet again, with a rapid decrease in estradiol, progesterone, and prolactin in the time following delivery. With this big change in hormones comes a significant change to the immune system. In the six months to a year following delivery, there's a boost in immune system activation, specifically in T cells, to protect you against viruses and infections. This time is also marked by changes to mood and mental health, with more than 50 percent of women experiencing postpartum blues. This is due to the rapid shift in hormones and significant decrease in serotonin production, and may even be related to changes in immune cell activity. Research shows that postpartum depression and psychosis may have to do with a lack of upregulation in the production of T cells, which leads to low-grade inflammation and sometimes even immune disorders such as postpartum thyroiditis.

From our experience with postpartum women, when started slowly, cold exposure can support mood, boost energy levels, and reduce stress during this time. The breathing exercises are another wonderful way to care for yourself and reduce pain and stress in this time of big feelings and physical recovery. During your pregnancy,

Isabelle: The WHM Basic Breathing exercise really helped me with the incision pain I experienced after giving birth. It turned out that my little one was happily eating himself to over nine pounds and was just a little bit too big to exit on his own. On day five after delivery, the pain was unbearable. With little sleep and in continuous pain, I felt so out of control of my body that when the midwife came to my house and told me they couldn't remove the stitches (it needed to be naturally resolved), tears streamed down my face. Later that day, I decided to do the Basic Breathing exercise again after having stopped for about eight months due to pregnancy. I lay down on the couch and after two rounds, suddenly I felt I was detaching from the pain. I could witness the sensation of pain without being absorbed by it. It was an exciting and almost spiritual moment, as the pain transformed into a wave of sensations going through my body. It's one thing when you repeatedly hear the WHM works for pain—it's another when you experience it! A perfect example of our motto of "feeling is understanding."

your breathing pattern likely changed, so now is the perfect time to focus on retraining your breath. It can take some time to readjust your breathing patterns, so this is a time when compassion and self-nurturing need to be your priority. Start with regular check-ins (refer to the steps on pages 91–92), observing what's going on in your body without pushing for things to be perfect—slowly but surely, your breathing will return to an optimal state. Depending on your mood and goal, you can choose one of several breathing techniques. The conscious breathing exercise (page 95) is a great choice; or, if you have a pelvic floor issue, check out the pelvic floor breathing exercise (pages 116–17). If you are dealing with pain or low mood, you can do the WHM Basic Breathing technique (pages 114–15).

Breastfeeding

Many women wonder if cold exposure will influence breastfeeding in a positive or negative way. Although this is a mostly unexplored area of research, our observation is that the short-term stress of cold exposure falls in the category of "healthy" stress versus the continuous stress that can be detrimental to milk production. Many women in the WHM community continue with cold exposure throughout their journey of breastfeeding. Always listen to your body, but if cold exposure helps you manage stress and boost your energy, then it's a healthy practice to incorporate during this phase.

It's wise to wait with cold exposure until your milk supply is fully up and running and you understand the feeding behavior of your

TESTIMONIAL: I actually started with Wim Hof's method because I suffered from various complaints during the menopause and nothing really seemed to help. I regularly experienced a tight feeling in my chest, often preceding a hot flash—a feeling of shortness of breath, which also brought feelings of panic and being trapped. However, when I started Wim Hof's cold water training, I discovered a surprising relief: when I step into the cold water of the lake, the tight and constricting feeling seems to slowly disappear. At a certain point my breathing becomes calm, and then it seems as if my lungs become very wide, as if something opens and I can absorb much more oxygen. This has a direct influence on my state of mind: suddenly I feel that everything will be fine and that in the end I can handle everything, no matter how difficult it may be. It is a feeling of serene strength that can sometimes linger for hours, even the following days. And then there is the remarkable effect the breathing exercise has on me. If I suffer from "brain fog" in the morning, the exercise quickly provides me with relief.

—Agnes

little one and your milk supply. For some women, breastfeeding happens easily, but for others, it takes some time. When you're ready, you can start with cold exposure and observe how the cold impacts it. Like most of our advice surrounding pregnancy and postpartum, don't stick to a rigid protocol, but instead incorporate the WHM in a compassionate and nurturing way. Start as if you were a beginner by ending your shower with ten to fifteen seconds—or even shorter— of cold, then build up in a way that feels good to you. If you are ready and planning to do more intense cold exposure, like ice bathing and cold nature dips, pay attention to timing. We don't recommend doing your cold exposure with breasts full of milk. If your breasts feel sensitive, you also might want to keep them out of the water.

PERIMENOPAUSE AND MENOPAUSE

"I don't feel like myself" or "What the f*ck is happening to me?" are phrases we often hear from women going through menopause, a time of great hormonal change. During the transition to menopause, called perimenopause, progesterone starts to decline, and estrogen, which has had a protective role in a woman's health all her life so far, starts to fluctuate in an erratic manner, leading to the symptoms often associated with menopause. As we learned in Chapter 3, estrogen is not only important for reproduction, but also vital for the heart and blood vessels, bones, breasts, skin, hair, mucous membranes, pelvic muscles, and brain, which explains why the symptoms of menopause extend to all parts of the body. And yet very little is available in terms of menopause research, support, and treatments. The transition into menopause can cause a range of daily symptoms that can last up to ten years. For most women, the symptoms associated with menopause arise between ages forty-five and fifty-six, but can happen as early as in the thirties, and may persist indefinitely. Statistics on menopause show that approximately 75 to 80 percent of women will experience hot flashes, night sweats, and heart palpitations. Other common symptoms are fatigue, sleep disturbances, brain fog, weight gain, insulin resistance, and high blood pressure. Up to 70 percent of women also experience psychological symptoms during this time, including anger, irritability, anxiety and tension, depression, loss of concentration, and loss of self-esteem and confidence.

Many women go through this hormonal transition thinking that they are going crazy and have to deal with it all by themselves. Women often feel misunderstood and dismissed by their physicians, who may refer them to specialists for individual symptoms or simply prescribe a pill—often with undesirable side effects—before sending them home. Have migraines? See a neurologist. Heart palpitations? Go to a cardiologist. Aches? Here's a painkiller. Sleep problems? Here's a prescription for sleeping pills. Many women report being diagnosed with depression, anxiety, ADHD, and more, only to later discover that their symptoms were related to menopause. Scientists also indicate that the symptoms have gotten twice as bad in the last fifty years. In 2024, Halle Berry made a now-famous plea to the US government to start funding menopause research, saying that we are missing so much knowledge about something that affects almost half of a woman's life! Welcome to the rabbit hole of menopause.

Put all this together, and the transition into menopause can leave many women desperately in need of practices to balance hormones, fight stress, and increase their resilience in the face of this big transition. Of course, this is where the WHM can really shine!

Stress and Inflammation

Cold exposure, breathing, and mindset shifts can greatly benefit women in menopause, as research shows that various menopause symptoms last longer and are more severe among women who are obese or stress-sensitive, deal with anxiety and depression, or have an existing hormonal or immune imbalance that's causing stress on the body. Stress can literally *steal* pregnenolone—the mother hormone that turns into progesterone, as cortisol is made from the same building blocks—and estrogen has been linked to more severe menopause symptoms. With the WHM, you can learn to stabilize your stress levels and to be more resilient during this transition phase. Some studies have established links between menopause symptoms and inflammation levels, and other studies have even described perimenopause as a "systemic inflammatory phase." Inflammation plays a key role in the chronic conditions that develop once women enter menopause, as the body is in a constant state of repair. Estrogen works as an anti-inflammatory and has a protective effect on the heart, cholesterol levels, and arterial health. When balanced, estrogen works to stimulate the immune system in healthy ways, but the unpredictable spikes and dips in estrogen during perimenopause can disrupt immune system balance. Menopause also greatly affects the gut microbiome balance, which is where a great deal of our immune system is located. As we know, the WHM can decrease inflammation and increase pro-inflammatory markers and may have immune-balancing effects.

Mood

An uptick in mood issues is extremely common during menopause. We know that feel-good hormones like serotonin, dopamine, adrenaline, and endorphins are all influenced by estrogen in one way or another. The brain is full of estrogen and progesterone receptors, and when our estrogen levels fluctuate or decline, it leaves women more vulnerable to depression, anxiety, and mood swings.

The WHM can tackle mood symptoms in menopause in many ways. It's been shown to reduce inflammation, which plays a major role in mental health. Anybody who's done cold exposure can attest to the instant mood-boosting effects. Research is extremely limited regarding women in menopause and cold exposure, but a great survey was published in 2024 supporting what thousands of women already experience and report. Of the 1,114 people who responded, 785 were perimenopausal and reported significant improvement in anxiety (46.9 percent), mood swings (34.5 percent), irritability (37.6 percent), and low mood (31.1 percent) with cold water swimming in nature. Even more interesting, 63.3 percent of the women reported that they swam specifically to reduce their hormonal symptoms.

Brain Fog

The WHM can bring instant alleviation to brain fog, which is a common issue for women going through perimenopause or menopause. This may be linked to how the method, especially the breathing exercises, promotes the movement of cerebrospinal fluid (CSF), which travels from the base of our spine all the way to the brain. Impaired sleep for women during perimenopause, due to the night sweats that keep them up, leads to a buildup of inflammation in the brain. Women especially need deep rest to make sure we properly restore our bodies, and one of the ways we do this is by clearing fluid. CSF can move quicker with the WHM breathing techniques. We liken it to a daily "brain shower," where we cleanse the buildup of toxins and waste products. We've heard many reports from women struggling from brain fog that the WMH brings them almost instant relief! We also know that cold exposure sharpens the mind, due to the noradrenaline boost.

Burnout, Energy, and Sleep

Fatigue and burnout are two major symptoms for women during menopause, and in recent years there has been an increase of menopause-related burnout. Increased energy is a major improvement women report when doing the WHM. The cold is also an undeniable energizer. Cold exposure in different forms leads to an increase of energy, increasing dopamine by 250 percent and nor-adrenaline 540 percent in one study. The beauty of the WHM for menopause-related burnout (and really any burnout for that matter) is its ability to work as a "chill pill" as well as an energizer, without the energy crash later on. Similarly, both cold exposure and inter-mittent hypoxia boost mitochondrial health, the energy factories of our cells. While the cold works as an instant energizer, together with the breathing exercises, we also activate the vagus nerve, re-setting the nervous system and activating our restorative function, which leads our body to reconnect with our circadian rhythm, allowing the natural urge to sleep to kick in.

Hot Flashes

The decline in estrogen during menopause is often accompanied by hot flashes, which are probably the most notorious symptom of menopause. The internal thermostat of women gets turned up, and in response, the body tries to cool off through hot flashes. About 75 percent of women experience hot flashes, and about 15 percent of women will experience severe hot flashes.

One study showed that women with moderate anxiety were nearly three times more likely to report hot flashes, and women with high anxiety were nearly five times more likely to report hot flashes. Women often report that stress triggers these hot flashes, so when we can improve our resilience to stress, we may also reduce hot flashes. Slow, deep breathing has also been touted as a great way to reduce hot flashes. One clinical trial showed a 42 to 52 percent decrease in hot flashes after just one or two fifteen-minute diaphragmatic breathing sessions per day. During these fifteen minutes, the women took six breaths per minute, and after just nine weeks, they saw these amazing benefits! In the survey mentioned before, the perimeno-pausal women who did cold water swimming also saw a 30.3 percent reduction in hot flashes.

By taking a cold shower, going into cold natural water, or even taking a short dip in an ice bath, we see many women greatly regulate their internal thermostat. There are many possible explanations, from the reduction in temperature itself to the constriction of veins, which may stop hot flashes from spreading.

Cardiovascular Health and Blood Pressure

When estrogen decreases during perimenopause, it can lead to a buildup of plaque in the arteries and contribute to the cardiovascular conditions, such as heart disease, stroke, and irregular heartbeats, that are common during this time in a woman's life. Psychological stress and sleep deprivation are strongly correlated with these issues, and reducing stress can lead to tremendous improvements.

With the breathing techniques, we can regulate our nervous system and stabilize our blood pressure and stress levels. Many women report decreasing their heart rate and blood pressure and increasing their heart rate variability practicing the method. As we learned in the chapter on cold exposure, the cold exercises the cardiovascular

A WORD OF CAUTION: There is a delicate dance between too much and too little cold exposure. For women with poor cardiovascular health, the system can be fragile. You need to do a very slow buildup, and not put too much strain on a system that is already strained. Ice baths for beginners with poor cardiovascular health or heart disease, or women who previously suffered a stroke should be started with caution, if at all, and always in consultation with your doctor. If you've been cleared by your doctor to be in a sauna or play sports, that's a sign ice baths might be safe for you as well. However, it is advisable to gradually experiment with cold exposure at more manageable temperatures, such as a cool shower.

system and flushes the arteries of this built-up plaque and fat and, more importantly, trains these little muscles in the veins to maintain their function.

Weight Gain and Insulin Resistance

Many women deal with weight gain and metabolic changes, such as high blood sugar and increased belly fat during menopause. Studies show that during the menopausal transition, women gain an average of one pound per year, and 20 percent of women gain ten pounds or more during these years, much of it accumulating in the midsection. This weight gain has many causes, but a major one is a decrease in insulin sensitivity that causes fat storage around the belly area. We know that acute cold exposure, such as an ice bath, will increase glucose uptake, activate brown fat, and increase insulin sensitivity. We know from studies on Wim that the intercostal muscles suck up glucose during cold exposure. One study showed that cold water swimming twice a week showed significant benefits for women's body composition and insulin sensitivity. Cold exposure also leads to the evolution of white fat to brown fat, which indicates a boost in metabolism. As you can see, several pathways have the potential to help menopausal women with insulin resistance and weight gain.

As women, we experience many transitions in life that can cause profound physical, emotional, and hormonal changes. While natural, they can significantly impact our sense of self, requiring adaptation to new physical realities and emotional landscapes. The WHM can help ease these transitions and promote quick and smooth adaptations to our ever-changing bodies.

THE WHM FOR INFLAMMATORY AND AUTOIMMUNE DISEASE

"Health is not only the absence of disease."

With new technologies, techniques, and treatments, modern medicine has made amazing strides in recent decades. Unfortunately, it still falls short when it comes to preventing and treating the chronic conditions that so many people struggle with. According to the Centers for Disease Control, 51.8 percent of US adults have at least one chronic health condition, and 27.2 percent have more than one. Nearly all these chronic diseases can be traced back to chronic inflammation.

You've probably heard about chronic inflammatory conditions like allergies, asthma, and arthritis, or autoimmune diseases like psoriatic arthritis, multiple sclerosis, and autoimmune thyroid disease. What you might not know is that inflammation is a root cause of the top causes of death and disability, including cardiovascular disease, stroke, chronic respiratory disease, cancer, diabetes, kidney disease, fatty liver disease, and neurodegenerative disorders like Alzheimer's disease. New scientific results even show that an imbalanced immune system and inflammatory response can lead to psychiatric diseases like depression, schizophrenia, postpartum psychosis, bipolar diseases, and autism. In one study, titled "Chronic Inflammation in the Etiology of Disease Across the Life Span," researchers explain that chronic systemic inflammation can lead to a variety of diseases that, together, represent the leading causes of disability and mortality worldwide. In fact, globally, three of five people die due to chronic inflammatory diseases, and 90 percent of Western diseases are immune-related.

The prevalence of both chronic inflammation and chronic health conditions is higher among women; women are nine times more likely to develop an autoimmune disease than men. Many people with these conditions struggle with constant symptoms, and medications can be helpful but also have their own risks and side effects. In fact, the number three cause of death worldwide is prescribed medication. To add insult to injury, research tells us that 80 percent of these chronic diseases are driven by lifestyle factors like stress, lack of exercise, nutrition, and smoking and drinking—all of which can be avoided with proper lifestyle practices.

As a result, all over the world, individual people are empowering themselves with knowledge about diet, lifestyle, and natural medicine to take back control over their own health. Women are leading this charge, experimenting with various modalities—like the WHM—when modern medicine falls short. Rather than tackling the symptoms, these modalities work to resolve the underlying issues of inflammation and autoimmunity. Our bodies have an incredible capacity to heal themselves; we just need to create the right conditions for that to happen, and the immune system is the best place to start.

WOMEN, INFLAMMATION, AND THE IMMUNE SYSTEM

You've probably thought about your immune system when you have a cold or the flu, but have you ever thought about where it's located? This intricate system is concentrated mostly in your lymph nodes and bone marrow, but it's also present in unexpected places, like your gut and even your ovaries. The immune system is big, making up a substantial percentage of your body's cells. In fact, if you weighed all the immune cells in an average-sized human—about 1.8 billion cells all together—they would weigh about 2.6 pounds, which is roughly the weight of a pineapple! Immune cells are so pivotal for survival that they are produced as early as three weeks after conception.

A healthy immune system strikes a balance between activation and suppression; it must activate quickly against threats like bacteria, injury, or toxins, but must also strike intelligently and accurately to avoid excessive activation, which can cause immune diseases and chronic inflammation. It must also know when to stand down, which allows it to focus on other functions, like repairing cellular damage or growing new tissues.

Unfortunately, as we've touched on in earlier chapters, our immune systems aren't always able to maintain this perfect balance, which can lead to chronic inflammation. Inflammation is an innate immune response to a threat, whether it's a foreign invader such as bacteria, virus, cancer, a transplanted organ, or even a psychological or emotional stressor. There are two types of inflammation. The good type is the body's acute response to microbes, tissue damage, metabolic stress, or any type of illness or injury. When the inflammatory response is short-term, it serves a very useful purpose by kick-starting our body's defense system, protecting against further damage and helping us to recover. The effects of acute inflammation can include pain, redness, swelling, and heat. Inflammation, in the short run, is a beautiful tool, as it allows the body to repair and heal.

PREVENTION—BOOST THE IMMUNE SYSTEM: Although this chapter dives into illnesses—where our immune system has failed to protect us or abandoned its role due to autoimmunity—we should point out that the method is also one of the best ways to prevent illness in the first place. It doesn't just help us manage illness, it helps us feel healthy and happy. Research shows that the WHM increases anti-inflammatory proteins and lowers pro-inflammatory proteins, indicating an all-around boost to the immune system. We've seen with our own eyes how everyday illnesses seem to fade into the shadows when you are regularly practicing the WHM. On the occasion that we do get sick, and get a flu, for example, the recovery time is often shockingly quick.

The bad kind of inflammation is chronic and low-grade, which involves a prolonged activation of the immune system. This type of inflammation might not cause noticeable symptoms right away, but the immune system is working overtime under the surface, and eventually, that will catch up to the body. As Professor Marcel Muskiet, an internal medicine physician and immune system expert, is quoted as saying: "We don't notice it, but constant low levels of inflammation are the breeding ground of many diseases."

Oftentimes, we are first made aware of this chronic inflammation when we develop an autoimmune disease. In this case, the immune system has suffered enough damage that it is unable to distinguish between real threats and the body's own tissues. It launches an attack against the body, which, over time, can lead to one of the more than eighty different autoimmune diseases. The specific mechanisms can vary depending on the type of disease, but chronic inflammation is often a common denominator, as it triggers and perpetuates the immune response against the body itself. This is called a loss of "tolerance."

As we mentioned earlier, women are nine times more likely to develop an autoimmune disease than men. The explanation for the massive gender gap is not fully understood. Although genetics is often cited as one of the main factors, it doesn't offer a complete explanation. Women do have a genetic predisposition for increased auto-antibodies, designed to protect their offspring from infection, but that may also increase the risk of an autoimmune disease. Other factors also play a role, including female sex hormones. Interestingly, the substantial increase in risk for autoimmune disease applies to women only during their reproductive years and seems to increase dramatically during times of great hormonal change, such as postpartum and in perimenopause. But when women enter menopause, the risk equalizes, which suggests that estrogen is a major contributor.

Interestingly, a strong correlation also exists between instances of autoimmune disease and periods of excessive stress. Retrospective studies have shown that up to 80 percent of patients with an autoimmune disease reported extreme emotional stress before their disease onset. The authors concluded, "It is presumed that the stress-triggered neuroendocrine hormones lead to immune dysregulation, which ultimately results in autoimmune disease, by altering or amplifying cytokine production."

WHAT ARE CYTOKINES? Cytokines are small proteins that play a crucial role in cell signaling. They act as messengers between cells, regulating immune responses and facilitating various physiological processes. Cytokines can have pro-inflammatory or anti-inflammatory effects and influence overall immune balance. Some common pro-inflammatory cytokines include IL-8, IL-6, and TNF-α. Excessive production of these cytokines contributes to chronic inflammation and a wide range of diseases. A lot of research on inflammation or inflammatory disease uses cytokines like TNF-α as a way to measure inflammation levels in the body.

As women, we should be conscious about this risk and, at the same time, remember that there are many ways to naturally support a healthy and balanced immune system, including the WHM.

THE WHM FOR CHRONIC INFLAMMATORY AND AUTOIMMUNE CONDITIONS

We recently attended a symposium on "The Future of Medicine," focused on autoimmune diseases and inflammation. One of the speakers, rheumatologist and immunologist Dr. Iain McInnes, highlighted TNF-alpha (TNF-α) as the master regulator of inflammation. When TNF-α is present, it indicates a high level of inflammation that needs to be managed. Inhibiting TNF-α has provided relief to people with various immune diseases—such as arthritis, psoriasis, inflammatory bowel disease, and others. This was a significant revelation, as it was identified as a factor that could potentially have a major impact on the future of medicine. Its crucial role in the onset of autoimmune diseases suggests it could be key to understanding and treating these conditions.

We were awestruck at hearing this! And our shock wasn't just at this new piece of information, but the fact that we already knew that the WHM has been linked to lower TNF-α levels. In fact, the famous Radboud study we've mentioned again and again throughout these chapters showed that the WHM lowered TNF-α by 53 percent and led to 33 percent reduction in pro-inflammatory markers IL-6 and IL-8 after just one session of WHM breathing after ten days of training in the WHM.

You would think that knowing all this, there would have been a surge of interest to conduct research on the WHM for chronic inflammation and autoimmune disease. If a "natural" pill could reduce inflammation by 33 to 50 percent with practically no potential negative side effects, as the WHM has shown, the company would make billions and could treat millions! But as our father always says, "Science is as slow as the slowest turtle," and there's a drastic lack of investment in natural healing methods regarding autoimmune conditions. Why? Our modern healthcare system does not focus on treating the root cause of an illness and incentivizes drugs, doctor visits, and more sickness—prioritizing profits instead of people. We know a lot of amazing doctors and researchers who want the best for people, but we also know their hands are often tied by insurance and pharmaceutical companies that don't want to lose their firm grip on the healthcare system. In fact, after the initial study, Radboud Medical University was motivated to do more research on the effect of the WHM on autoimmune diseases, but it was tremendously difficult to gain funding to support studies on any type of natural healing modality. The university wanted to do the study on arthritis, which is a common inflammatory condition affecting women, but the Reumafonds—a fund specifically created to invest in research on rheumatism—declined their request for funding, even after recognizing that the Wim Hof Method does show promise for this disease.

Luckily, science is slowly catching up. We are starting to see more nutrition, stress reduction, and lifestyle advice in doctors' offices. In the Netherlands, nature walks are even prescribed as a form of medicine. We are also starting to see research published on the WHM and chronic inflammatory and autoimmune diseases. For many years now, we have been working with various scientific and medical institutions to conduct research into the WHM for chronic diseases—with promising results!

Arthritis

After many slow years, another study was finally conducted to test the effects of the WHM on people with autoimmune disease. The research was a collaboration with Amsterdam Medical University under the lead of Professor Geert Buijze. Dr. Buijze is a neurosurgeon and has always been very interested in studying the WHM; years before, he joined Wim's Kilimanjaro trip and wrote a paper showing that the WHM was effective in combating acute mountain sickness after the experience.

The researchers tested the WHM as an add-on intervention to the participants' current treatment for axial spondylarthritis, a type of inflammatory arthritis that mostly affects the lower back, hips, and buttocks. This specific autoimmune disease was chosen because it affects relatively young people who have fewer comorbidities, which makes the results more clear-cut. The participants practiced the method daily for eight weeks. The training consisted of breathing exercises, weekly whole-body ice baths (incrementally for a maximum of five minutes), daily cold showers (incrementally up to two and a half minutes), and a type of interoceptive meditation. Incredibly, when compared to a control group, the "Hof group" experienced significant declines in at least three measurements of inflammation in the body and also showed increases in quality-of-life scores and significant physical improvements. The authors suggested the WHM is a promising "novel therapeutic approach in patients with inflammatory conditions."

The results of this follow-up research helped get more research off the ground, and studies were conducted on the WHM and other chronic health conditions.

Psoriasis

Psoriasis affects about 4 percent of the population and causes dry, itchy, scaly patches on the skin, oftentimes on the knees, elbows, and scalp. Psoriasis is considered an immune condition, as the dry patches are due to the immune system producing new cells in an overly accelerated way. Currently there are treatments for psoriasis, but no cure.

According to the National Psoriasis Foundation, stress is one of the most common psoriasis triggers, so it won't come as a surprise that we have heard countless anecdotal stories of people in our community improving their psoriasis with the WHM. These stories motivated Dr. Jan Czarnecki, at the Institute of Psychiatry and Neurology at the Medical University of Lodz, to run a clinical trial investigating the effect of the WHM on psoriasis.

For this trial, half of the thirty-eight participants with psoriasis did ten weeks of training, consisting of breathing exercises, cold exposure, and meditation, while the other half maintained their typical treatment. The researchers took blood and saliva samples throughout and closely monitored the skin condition with questionnaires and evaluations. In a bit of a plot twist, two weeks after the intervention there was a full lockdown due to the COVID-19 pandemic, which added a lot of stress to the shoulders of the participants. The results showed flare-ups were more prevalent among the control group, with 55 percent of the control group participants reporting an increase in their usage of topical treatments. This result was confirmed by a saliva test that showed an increase in inflammation markers and a decrease in anti-inflammatory markers. In the intervention group, a slight improvement in the condition was observed, with 68 percent of the subjects reporting a reduction in topical treatment usage. This was confirmed by a saliva test, showing decreased levels of inflammatory cytokines. The Dermatology Life Quality Index also improved fourfold in the intervention group, with improved sleep quality, reduced depressive symptoms, and increased mindfulness.

Endometriosis

Endometriosis is a poorly understood condition that affects around 15 percent of women in their reproductive years. With endometriosis, uterine-like tissue grows outside the uterus, leading to inflammation and scar tissue, mostly in the pelvic area. Endometriosis can cause severe pain and contribute to infertility. Sometimes, surgery is even needed to remove the tissue. For years, this condition has been misdiagnosed and sometimes not taken seriously, with many doctors brushing it off as simply part of a woman's normal monthly hormonal fluctuations. Recently, due to a lot of advocating from women, more research and funding has gone into understanding this condition.

The first time we heard that the WHM could possibly benefit endometriosis was through the wife of Dr. Nigel Beach, a physiotherapist who later became a certified WHM instructor. He and his wife had both been practicing the method, and he came to my father one day and said that after practicing the WHM, his wife, who had been struggling with fertility, got pregnant. (They even gave their child the middle name Wim!) Dr. Beach pushed the University of Waikato to conduct research on the method back in 2017. (Unfortunately, it never came to fruition because of—once again—lack of funding.) Luckily, in 2023, Wim met a couple while strolling on the beach in Australia. The wife, who had endometriosis, became highly motivated to research the WHM and its potential effects on endometriosis after hearing Wim speak. They just happened to be philanthropists and ended up funding a study on the WHM and endometriosis that is currently underway. Until we know more, we can hypothesize that the WHM may be effective against endometriosis because of its ability to suppress inflammation; previous research has shown us that there is a clear link between inflammation and endometriosis, especially the inflammatory cytokines IL-6 and TNF-α, which the WHM is already known to target. Like most other chronic illnesses, inflammation is at the root of endometriosis. This overlap makes this area of study extremely promising, especially for a disease that leaves women with few good treatment options.

TESTIMONIAL: I was diagnosed with endometriosis when I was twenty-eight years old. I had been having pain for months when going to the bathroom, which I first thought might be due to something in my diet, but then I started to feel new and more severe pain during my period as well as pain during intercourse. When I asked my gynecologist about it on my next visit, he told me it was endometriosis; he explained that doctors didn't really know the cause of the disease, but that many women get it and that there is a connection to high levels of stress. I was definitely going through quite a bit of stress in work and life at the time. I am a high-performing person, and at that time, I was managing a very important project and also dealing with some personal matters. Given my symptoms, my doctor scheduled me for an operation that would take place in a few months. During those months, I started practicing the Wim Hof Method. Not necessarily because of the endometriosis but because I met my now husband, who is a WHM instructor. Almost every day I did the cold exposure, breathing, and mindset practices, and I loved how it taught me to be more present in the face of challenges. I learned to find the feeling of peace in the ice bath and then carry it with me back into the world, which had a profound impact on me. After a few months, I went back to my gynecologist for a check-in before the operation. When he examined me, there was no sign of endometriosis whatsoever. Everything was gone, so he canceled the operation. It was obvious to me and my doctor that since I had found balance mentally, my body found its way back to balance as well.

—Tanit

These studies have given us positive early results that display the incredible benefits of the WHM and establish a foundation for research to continue to build on top of. Hopefully in the coming years, there will be dozens of studies on the WHM for various chronic health conditions. That said, we can't wait for science to catch up. Our father loves science and scientists, but he never let the lack of science or funding for research dictate what he could do and teach. By its very nature, science is reductionist. It's meant to test specific and isolated phenomena, not to describe the vast realm of all possibilities under the sun. Science is much like the ocean or space—we only know so much, and we need to keep exploring and experimenting.

As our father says, "my body is my laboratory." New frontiers can only be discovered when we are open to exploring and trying new things. And what many women have discovered in their personal laboratory is that alternative therapies like the Wim Hof Method can be incredibly healing when it comes to their unique health challenges. Women are leading this charge, experimenting with various modalities—with great success—when their own physicians or the healthcare system fall short. We have witnessed thousands of women suffering from the following chronic illnesses find relief through the Wim Hof Method.

Polycystic Ovary Syndrome

Polycystic ovary syndrome (PCOS) is a hormonal condition affecting a whopping 8 to 13 percent—with some sources saying it may be as high as 20 percent—of women during their reproductive years. If you have this condition, you may struggle with irregular periods, excess androgen levels that cause acne, male pattern hair growth, hair thinning, weight gain, mood swings, and cysts in the ovaries. Irregular periods, which are usually accompanied by a lack of ovulation, can make it difficult to become pregnant, making PCOS the leading cause of female infertility. PCOS is also linked to increased risk of depression, cancer, heart disease, and stroke, especially for women in perimenopause.

Like many hormone conditions, there's still a lot we don't know about how to prevent, diagnose, and treat PCOS. What we do know is that insulin resistance, inflammation, genetics, high cortisol, and imbalanced hormone levels all play a role in the onset of this condition. We have seen many women treat symptoms of PCOS with the WHM. The breathing exercises, cold exposure, and mindset shifts also seem to help with the underlying issues causing PCOS in the long term, sometimes leading to the lessening of the condition overall.

Thyroid Disease and Hashimoto's

An important part of the neuroendocrine system, the thyroid gland is responsible for many different functions in the body, such as metabolism, thermoregulation, and even regulation of the immune system. In the hierarchy of hormones, cortisol—which is in charge of survival—rules over the thyroid and the reproductive hormones, which are in charge of less vital functions like metabolism and reproduction. This is an intelligent design, but the chronic stress of our modern world can cause constant cortisol production, which wreaks havoc on our thyroid health.

The most common thyroid condition is Hashimoto's, an autoimmune condition that causes an underproduction of thyroid hormone. People with this condition often report feeling weak and tired and often struggle with muscle pain and depression. Like most of the conditions in this chapter, stress plays a big role in Hashimoto's, with one study showing that a stress management program for women with Hashimoto's reduced feelings of depression and anxiety. Women are four to ten times more likely than men to develop Hashimoto's, and it seems to be triggered most often during big hormonal transitions like puberty, pregnancy, and perimenopause.

We have seen many women manage their thyroid conditions with the Wim Hof Method. That said, Hashimoto's disease can also cause increased cold sensitivity, so we always recommend a gentle approach to cold exposure, starting with a cold rinse at the end of a warm shower. The pain receptors can be so sensitive when we experience more stress in our bodies, and a little cold can already be so energy-draining that any stressor needs to be added with full cooperation between mind and body. In these instances, less is more, so make sure you don't go past the point where it drains you of energy. If you find yourself low on energy, take it easy and listen to your body. Just like a newbie in the gym won't lift a hundred-pound dumbbell, you'll have to build up your strength and energy.

If you're using the WHM for Hashimoto's, we also recommend focusing on nose breathing and lengthening the exhales during the breathing practices, since Hashimoto's can put us into a hypervigilant state and may benefit from increased activation of the vagus nerve and parasympathetic nervous system.

Chronic Pain and Fibromyalgia

Wim once received a personal message from a woman who, until she found the WHM, had chronic pain so severe she had wanted to end her own life. Luckily, she found great relief with the method and wanted to thank Wim for bringing the hope and spirit back into her life.

Chronic pain affects the lives of millions. In the US alone, an estimated 20.9 percent of adults have chronic pain. Research indicates that alongside heightened sensitivity to temperature, women also exhibit increased sensitivity to pain. This is attributed to their higher nerve density, which amplifies their perception of external stimuli, making women more responsive to their surroundings.

Scientific studies on the WHM also point to its painkilling effects. Radboud Medical University showed that the WHM was effective at increasing pain tolerance not only right after the session, but for a period of hours after, which could go a long way toward making pain more manageable. There are many possible ways the WHM fights off pain: for one, the huge release of adrenaline, beta-endorphins, and noradrenaline, which are known to have pain-relieving and mood-boosting effects. Some research suggests that the WHM may activate compounds called "endogenous" opioids and cannabinoids. "Endogenous" means produced inside an organism or cell, and these compounds are essentially our body's naturally produced version of opioid painkillers or cannabinoids, which include compounds found in cannabis, like CBD and THC.

The WHM also fights off inflammation, which is a root cause of chronic pain. One example of this is the chronic musculoskeletal disorder fibromyalgia, which causes pain all over the body. Between 80 to 96 percent of people with this condition are women, and studies show women experience more severe pain from the condition than men. For a long time, the cause of fibromyalgia was unknown, but recent research revealed that inflammation, especially inflammatory markers IL-6 and IL-8—which are also targeted by the WHM—are strongly linked to fibromyalgia. We have seen women find great relief from fibromyalgia symptoms by practicing the method.

Cancer

While there's very limited research, early reports show that the WHM may be beneficial in the prevention of cancer and could potentially be used as an add-on treatment to complement traditional cancer therapy. A big part of this lies in the WHM's ability to target stress, which has been connected to an increased risk for cancer in some studies. In fact, as much as 42 percent of women report that instances of malignancy of breast cancer are linked with a major emotional stressor in their lives. Emotional stress has a severe impact on physical reality, and the method can intercept a cycle of stress and disease. As Professor Pierre Capel underlines in his book *The Emotional DNA*, psychological stress—but also psychological intervention—can have a direct effect on the course of a disease like breast cancer. Oxytocin, a social-bonding hormone that is released during relaxation, has been shown to have a cancer-fighting effect. The WHM may also bring balance back to inflammation levels and the immune system, which also have a role to play in cancer prevention and treatment. Other hypotheses that need more study include increasing blood flow and cardiovascular health, aiding with lymphatic drainage, and temporarily altering internal pH.

We do have one study on the connection between the cold and cancer to draw more firm conclusions from. In 2022, the leading scientific journal *Nature* published a study on mice showing that during cold exposure, their brown fat consumed more glucose. This might not seem directly related to cancer, but research shows that glucose is critical to cancer growth and development, acting as the fuel cancer uses to grow and spread. The researchers observed that cold exposure "arrests tumor progression" by 80 percent at a room temperature of 39.2 degrees, through the activation of brown fat metabolism and glucose starvation. Similar results were shown in a pilot study on an eighteen-year-old patient with lymphoma. This patient had undergone five chemotherapy sessions and still had active tumors. After a mere seven days of exposure to a 71.6-degree environment, which isn't even uncomfortably cold, the patient's tumor cells had a significantly reduced glucose uptake. This area of research is in very early stages but suggests cold exposure may represent a simple but novel treatment method.

In our years of teaching the WHM, we have seen this promising area of treatment firsthand. We've had women share stories of breast lumps decreasing and white cells increasing—which is necessary to be able to undergo chemotherapy safely—and many of these women are steadfast that the method had a big role to play in their improvement. They often share that their doctors were stunned at their progress and asked if they were doing anything differently, to which they answered: the Wim Hof Method. Because of this, we have engaged in many discussions with hospitals and doctors who have shown strong interest in conducting a study on the WHM for people with cancer. However, this type of research is particularly sensitive, and challenges such as funding shortages or negative feedback from ethical review boards have, so far, stalled these conversations.

If you're practicing the WHM for a chronic health condition, we recommend performing the breathing exercises every morning. When you have a health condition, especially one based on inflammation, you need to support your body's healing daily. That said, many people with a chronic condition also suffer from extreme lack of energy or chronic pain or other symptoms, so we always say to make sure that you experiment with cold exposure gradually, listen to your body, and never force it. When you have a chronic disease, you need to listen to not only the aches and pains, but also the emotions you feel.

THE WHM AND CHRONIC DISEASE— RECONNECTING THE BODY AND BRAIN

Any health condition—from cancer to PCOS to psoriasis—can make us feel disconnected from our body. Your symptoms may make you feel angry, out of control, or like a victim of your body. It's in healing these emotional hardships that we think the WHM has limitless potential. The breathing, cold, and mindset shifts have an amazing ability to bring you back to your body and allow you to reconnect. The cold can be empowering because it reconnects you with your body, allowing you to regain control in a moment of intense stress, and really let go of the crap that's holding you back. This shift in mindset is transformative, instilling the belief that you can influence your health, even when it feels like you've lost control. You are in control—not the disease.

This incredible transformation can be explained by more than just mindset shifts.

The anti-inflammatory benefits of the WHM don't just affect physical conditions, they may also improve our mental health. In fact, there's an entire field of study called immuno-neuroendocrinology. Dr. Hemmo Drexhage, an emeritus professor in medical immunology at Erasmus University Medical Center in the Netherlands, has been researching the interplay between our immune systems and the structure and function of the brain, mood, and behavior. He is the coordinator of Mood Stratification, a multinational research project investigating how our immune system determines abnormal mood and behavior. In his book *Immuno-Psychiatrie*, he explains just how interconnected the immune system, hormonal system, and brain are. When we are in a state of constant fight-or-flight, cortisol rises, while parts of the immune system are activated and other parts are downregulated. This results in feelings of burnout and a higher risk of infection and metabolic dysregulation. When the immune system is intrinsically faulty, it ages prematurely and the immune cells in the brain (called microglia) do not execute their normal function anymore, which is the buildup and functional regulation of those parts of the brain that coordinate our mood and behavior under stress. This results in abnormal moody and behavioral reactions to even light forms of stress. The prematurely aging immune system is also a risk factor for infections and autoimmune diseases. In fact, previous research has already shown that autoimmunity increases the likelihood of having conditions like depression, schizophrenia, bipolar disorder, or autism. This deeply intertwined relationship between the immune system and the brain is becoming clearer by the day. In the next chapter, we'll dive deeper into mental health and how the WHM can support mood and well-being on a psychological level.

THE WHM FOR MENTAL HEALTH

"Let go of what is too heavy to carry."

Our mother suffered from severe mental health issues that resulted in her ending her own life. The severe trauma from that is part of what inspired our father to deepen his practice with breathing, mindset, and going into the cold. These practices—which our father did on his own for years, and which he credits with helping him recover from this trauma—are what would eventually become the WHM. Today, we have seen thousands of people use the method to support their mental health with great success.

This is especially critical for women, who—like in the case of inflammatory conditions and chronic stress—disproportionately suffer from mental illness compared to men. In fact, anxiety and depression rates are twice as high in women, and we are at higher risk for other disorders such as bipolar disorder, post-traumatic stress disorder (PTSD), schizophrenia, and obsessive-compulsive disorder (OCD).

Why is this? We're still learning about the underlying causes of the modern mental health crisis, and why women are at higher risk than men. We know that major life stressors can trigger depression and anxiety, and research shows a strong link between female hormonal transitions—such as during puberty, the premenstrual phase, postpartum, and perimenopause and menopause—and rates of depression and anxiety, psychosis, mania, suicide attempts, and alcohol use.

We also know there is a balance of genetic and environmental factors at play. Each of us has a set of genes that create a baseline risk for mental health issues. Scientists used to think that these genes predetermined us to disease or not, but now we know that what we do and experience during life can have just as much—if not more—of an impact. You can think of it as an individual stress signature that is very personal to each of us; a signature that can literally turn on or off genes related to mental health issues. For example, you may have a genetic predisposition to depression, but if you are not exposed to stressful life events, that gene may never get turned on.

One notable risk factor is adverse childhood experiences (ACEs), which include things like experiencing or witnessing violence, abuse, or neglect as children. We know that women experience more traumatic events in their life on average, and that trauma tends to also leave a bigger negative imprint on our brains, with research showing women suffer more frequently from post-traumatic stress disorder (PTSD) than men with similar traumatic backgrounds. Women are more trigger-sensitive and have a higher tendency for dissociation, which is a mental process where a person disconnects from the world around them and their own brain, body, and memories, and sometimes even their identity. Women are also more prone to being hit with multiple triggers, stressors, and traumas all at once, with little to no recovery time in between. Over time, this will leave a big mark. As Dr. Stanley Rosenberg, the author of the book *Accessing the Healing Power of the Vagus Nerve*, wrote: "Ideally, we should be able to reset our nervous system and get a fresh start [after a traumatic event, but] . . . the effects of the traumatic events [can] stick with us long after the original shock."

When we can't recover from stressful or traumatic events, our stress response can become maladaptive. As a result, cortisol can rise quickly and erratically, and stay elevated for prolonged periods, while the amygdala—our fear center—grows and becomes more activated and more easily triggered. At the same time, the hippocampus, which plays a role in memory formation and linking emotions to memories, will shrink. Put all this together and we will no longer accurately assess the stressors we encounter daily; instead, our alarm system will go off at even the slightest trigger. This can create a loop of more stress and lead to various negative outcomes, including not just mental health issues but also physical health issues. In one example, studies show that women with PTSD have twice the risk for ovarian cancer and 71.5 percent of women with fibromyalgia suffer from PTSD.

We can learn to process past trauma and deal with chronic stress, change our stress signature, and increase our potential for emotional regulation for the better, both short- and long-term. The brain is always changing, a process called neuroplasticity, and we can play a big role in redirecting its growth.

THE WHM FOR MENTAL HEALTH

The researchers of the 2018 "Brain over Body" study underlined that "the practice of the Wim Hof Method (WHM) might allow practitioners to develop a higher level of control over key components of the autonomous system related to mood regulation." The researchers concluded that these remarkable results could have massive implications for multiple illnesses, including those related to mental health.

The WHM provides a format for processing our emotions, combating chronic stress, and releasing trauma. As instructors, we witness complete mental transformations in every single workshop or training session. We guide women through a thirty-minute breathing session, and a two-minute ice bath, and we shift their mindset. They leave, completely transformed, in under four hours. Can it be that simple? Yes, it can! Try sitting in an ice bath for two minutes while thinking about your problems. You can't. The issues you're dealing with and accompanying rumination disappear during the process, mental clouds fade away, and clarity and newfound resolve emerge.

So many people turn to the Wim Hof Method to help with mental health issues like depression, anxiety, and trauma, or even loss of purpose, low self-esteem, addiction, and burnout. We often hear that the WHM gave them a newfound sense of control, like they finally had something to say in the matter of their mental health; that it gave them back hope and the belief that things can get better. When they keep practicing in the long term, we often witness their entire lives change. We have received countless letters and messages of gratitude and have had many people come back to retreats wanting to tell us about their mental health healing in person, and each example shows how powerful the WHM is for mental health.

It's not just personal stories that showcase the WHM's mental health benefits; we also have quite a bit of science to support the dramatic transformations we witness at every workshop and retreat. We now have various studies into the WHM that unravel the mechanisms that lie underneath its effectiveness for mood regulation and mental health.

Mood and Emotional Regulation

One of the first studies on the WHM on mental health was a retrospective study in collaboration with Professor Marc Cohen of the Royal Melbourne Institute of Technology (RMIT) University in

Australia. This 2017 study, which took the form of a questionnaire, included data from more than 3,200 "Hoffers" (by this time, Wim Hof Method practitioners had already developed a nickname). This large sample size gave us enough data to gain a high-level understanding of the benefits people practicing the method were reporting. The results showed that people practicing the method reported less stress, less anxiety and depression, and improved mood, as well as improved mental focus and insomnia. In fact, approximately two-thirds of the 3,200 people reported significant mood improvements.

In 2023, researchers at the University of Michigan Medical School, led by Professor Vaibhav Diwadkar, hoped to uncover the mechanisms behind the WHM's benefits. Participants underwent a six-week WHM training that involved breathing exercises and cold exposure in the form of cold showers and ice baths. They used an fMRI device to scan the activity of the brain, looking specifically at the impact of the training on the endocannabinoid system.

THE ENDOCANNABINOID SYSTEM: This system is a complex cell-signaling system found in all vertebrates. It plays a crucial role in maintaining homeostasis in the body. In a healthy brain, the endocannabinoid system helps maintain a stable emotional state, preventing excessive anxiety and acting as a buffer against stress. The endocannabinoid system involves a series of natural compounds and receptors that are located all over the body. One type of receptor, called a cannabinoid-type 1 (CB1) receptor, is widespread in the brain and acts as a stress response buffer and regulator.

The study found that the WHM led to substantial increases in CB1 receptor binding across the brain. Increases in the activity of this receptor are strongly correlated with improved resilience to stress, mood, and anxiety. After the six-week WHM practice, participants also showed significantly lower anxiety and depressive symptoms, and those with the greatest increase in CB1 receptor activity saw the most mental health improvements. According to the researchers, the release of endocannabinoids might be a signature effect of the WHM. They even concluded that a "relatively short six-week WHM intervention positively impacts brain markers that have been associated with stress resistance, mood, anxiety and interoceptive function." Interestingly, the endocannabinoid system is also connected to the immune system, and the activation of cannabinoid receptors can switch the brain's immune cells, called microglial cells, into a more restorative and healing state.

A few years earlier, a study was conducted in collaboration with the University of California San Francisco (UCSF) to investigate the impact of the WHM on mood in female participants. Led by Dr. Elissa Epel, one of the most renowned and experienced researchers in the field of stress, the research team observed 141 women as they practiced the WHM (in the form of cold showers and WHM breathing exercises) and compared them to groups who did HIIT workouts, meditation, or slow-paced breathing every single day.

After three weeks, the WHM group showed similar decreases in stress and depression to the HIIT group but had even larger improvements in mood than the HIIT group. Results also showed that the WHM group reported more positive emotions than the other groups and continued to have more positivity in their lives three months later. And this is all with just cold showers! We would love to reproduce this study with our beloved ice baths, which are even more powerful.

Depression

We all have down days where we feel low in our mood, energy, and motivation, but depression is much more severe and long-lasting than just a day or two, and can influence how you think, feel, act, and perceive the world around you for months or years on end. People with depression have ongoing sadness, loss of interest in pleasurable things, fatigue, problems concentrating, and may also have thoughts of suicide. About one in three (29 percent) adults suffer from depression at one point in their lives, and women are about twice as likely to suffer from depression than men.

There are many underlying causes of depression. There is a known genetic factor, and there's a strong link between trauma and depression risk. Someone who has had four or more traumatic events in their childhoods is 450 percent more likely to develop depression and has a 1,200 percent higher chance of being suicidal. There is also an interesting connection between inflammation and depression. We remember that when the Radboud endotoxin study in 2014 was just published, a psychiatrist approached us who was interested in studying the WHM for people with depression due to its ability to target inflammatory markers. We designed the training protocol, and she wrote the proposal for the study and applied for funding, but it was denied. In recent years, however, this relationship has become too obvious to ignore. In 2023, the UK Biobank biomedical database published data revealing that people with depressive episodes have significantly higher levels of inflammatory cytokines in their blood. It was also found that a quarter of people who are depressed have evidence of low-grade inflammation in the blood. It seems that depression is related especially to an increase in IL-6, a cytokine we already know is targeted by the WHM. Interestingly, IL-6 also causes symptoms of everyday acute sicknesses like the flu, which may explain some of the overlap in symptoms with depression, such as reduced appetite, diminished social interest, and low sex drive.

Of the over 3,200 people who participated in the big RMIT survey, 722 reported a history of depression. Of those 722 respondents, 619 mentioned that practicing the WHM helped them somewhat to completely cure their depression. One case study on a twenty-four-year-old woman showed that a protocol of cold exposure led to a gradual reduction in her depression symptoms that was so significant, she was able to get off her medication. At the one-year follow-up, the benefits have persisted. A study done on the WHM for people with mild depression in collaboration with UCSF also showed it lowered depression; this study's full results are not yet available, but the benefits we've seen of the WHM for depression point in a very hopeful direction, and it's proving to be a powerful method for those suffering with this mental disorder. In our community, we have many people report that the WHM helped them alleviate or even overcome their depression entirely.

TESTIMONIAL: After my first child was born, I fell into postpartum depression without even realizing it. Being a first-time mom is a heavy burden on its own, let alone being the mother of a newborn who doesn't sleep. My daughter woke up approximately ten times per night until she was almost two years old. Coupled with her desire to explore the world faster than her body would allow, it drained my energy, and I felt like I was in a fog for quite a long time after her birth. When my second child was born, I knew what to expect. I allowed myself to rest for three months and focus on just being with the baby, but after that, I knew I had to take action to avoid falling into depression again. That's when I came across the Wim Hof Method, which piqued my interest. I started with cold showers. As someone who really dislikes the cold, the feeling after the shower came as a complete surprise—I felt rejuvenated, gained clarity, and, most importantly, was able to establish a calmness and energy for my baby. From that point on, I took a cold shower every morning, followed by some stretching and the horsestance to warm myself up. Mind you, I started this practice in the middle of winter—not the easiest time to begin cold showers!

When my baby was seven months old, I discovered that we had a certified Wim Hof Method instructor in our country, and within three days, I was attending her workshop. Understanding the importance of breathing opened up a new dimension of the Wim Hof practice for me. I began incorporating breathing exercises along with cold exposure, transitioning from cold showers at home to immersing myself in cold water in nature. It's fascinating how, with the help of the Wim Hof Method, I managed to calm my nervous system, even though I was physically exhausted. I cannot begin to explain how much better I felt after my second birth compared to my first. There were no signs of depression, I managed to maintain my energy levels, and I was present and calm for my baby. My second child is now two years old, and the Wim Hof Method is still my go-to remedy for any challenges that might compromise my mental well-being.

—Ursula

Anxiety

We can all feel anxious about an anticipated event or situation in life. When we feel anxious, it's our body communicating to us that something doesn't feel safe, be it imaginary or real. This signal translates into a feeling of uneasiness, worry, or nervousness. Physically, you tighten up, and your heartbeat and breathing rate can go up. For some people, anxious feelings play a major role in their life; many are completely overwhelmed by these feelings and their fear starts to dominate their behavior, and they may be diagnosed with an anxiety disorder, such as a panic disorder, social anxiety disorder, or a phobia. These disorders can evoke sudden intense feelings of anxiety and fear that are difficult to regulate and keep in proportion with the actual situation. Just like depression, women are twice as likely to suffer from an anxiety disorder compared to men.

The causes of anxiety are not fully understood, but genetic factors and past trauma appear to be major contributors as well as certain medical conditions, such as thyroid issues or blood sugar issues or heart disease. The WHM can benefit people with anxiety in many ways. The RMIT survey showed that one of the top positive results of practicing the WHM was a reduction in anxiety. Out of 826 people mentioning they had anxiety, 90 percent reported a positive impact on anxiety levels. People often report being more at peace and less tense and threatened by situations immediately after practicing the method. By not spending time on worry or rumination, we can preserve our energy to get the most out of our lives. When we do hard things and grow as a person, we restore our belief in ourselves and our trust in the world.

Trauma

Painful emotions need to be felt, or they will be stored in the body and brain. This is why, when it's not processed properly, trauma tends to reveal itself years later. This is common in childhood trauma, as children going through multiple traumatic events often block them out, only to have them come back up again in their thirties and forties in the form of mental or physical health issues. A 1990 study by the CDC showed that childhood trauma dramatically increases the risk of anxiety and depression as well as seven out of ten of the leading causes of death. Trauma can affect the development of the brain, the immune system, and even our DNA. Trauma can triple the risk for heart disease and lung cancer. And it's not only childhood trauma. Traumatic events can occur in any phase of life and threaten our emotional, mental, and physical well-being. On average, women experience more trauma in life than men, and marginalized groups are at an even higher risk.

For us to deal with trauma, the first thing we need to do is feel safe in our environment and in our bodies, before we can even start connecting to our emotions. As Dr. Gabor Maté says, we need to feel safe to be able to finally feel what it is we need to release. When we feel safe in our environment, then we can start doing internal work and connecting with emotions stored within us. This enables us to freely cry, scream, or unleash whatever comes up while we connect deeply with stored emotions. In our workshops and trainings, we see so many people who have lived for so long in a constant state of stress that they haven't been able to connect with their emotions, and some have not cried for years. During the process and in the safe space that we create, many of them finally get in touch with these emotions that have been ignored or blocked.

In 2023, the largest randomized controlled study on the WHM was done in collaboration with the University of Queensland. It involved a group of 404 participants (more than 50 percent were women) who were divided into a group that did WHM in-person instruction with ice baths, one that did WHM online instruction with cold showers, and one that did a mindful awareness-based meditation for four weeks. Both groups practicing the Wim Hof Method showed statistically significant improvements in various mental, psychological, and physical health indicators. Interestingly, feelings of psychological safety also improved in the WHM groups. Psychological safety is a measure of one's relationship to their environment and tells us that the WHM participants were able to let their guard down and really feel without fear of judgment.

It's not uncommon for people to break down, cry, and get in touch with painful periods in their life. They finally process childhood events, their divorce, or the loss of a loved one after years of suppressing their feelings. These are often the most beautiful moments because right then and there, the person made a huge leap in the healing process. While most of the participants of this study were male, the finding

of a recent study showed that after just one WHM-inspired intervention, participants reported a 37.5 percent reduction in unwanted
memories. After one month of practicing the WHM, a 50 percent
reduction was observed. The vividness and emotional intensity of the
memories was significantly reduced.

Laura: I cry almost every breathing session out of gratitude,
as I let go of my own stored-up emotions. Feeling my feelings
becomes so easy when we do the breathing exercises, and even
easier after having done the ice bath because it removes all of
your protective layers and makes you more vulnerable. Stored
emotions tend to rise when we feel comfortable enough to let
them out in a safe setting, and the WHM provides the perfect
setting for us to feel, while being heart-centered and full of
compassion and love for ourselves, which is the condition to
love others.

Trauma is at the root of many physical, mental, and emotional
challenges. Time and time again, we see that the method brings
people past the conditioned mind and allows them to access deep
layers of their subconscious where trauma can be dealt with. Sometimes, there is an instant feeling of empowerment, and sometimes,
it can unleash a lot of emotions that need to be combed through.
Almost everybody will experience a moment where they will cry
and release whatever needs to be released. But when we deal with
trauma, we deal with the root cause of so many mental health issues
in our lives.

We will always carry our mom in our hearts and beings, and we
have used the very tools in this book to release our own emotions,
heal, and continue forward with clarity, presence, gratitude, and joy.

Life offers countless ways to be lived, yet one truth remains clear: it's a miracle that we are here, and it's a miracle that we can fully experience everything within and around us. As Wim often says: "I am not afraid to die, I am afraid to not live life fully." The Wim Hof Method is a powerful tool that helps us shape our inner world, allowing us to perceive life more vividly and witness its unfolding with more ease.

BIOHACK WITH THE WHM: LONGEVITY AND THE FEMALE CYCLE

The Wim Hof Method is often categorized as a wellness practice, and has been embraced by the mindfulness, yoga, and beauty industries. But it's also being embraced by the medical, biohacking, sports, and even mountaineering worlds. In these contexts, the WHM is often praised for its possible longevity benefits by professional athletes and biohackers alike.

Longevity is an area of scientific research gaining a lot of traction in recent years. For one, life expectancy has increased dramatically since 1900, when the average lifespan was 47 years, compared to today, when people can expect to live to an average of 77.5 years. This is a massive change in a short period of time and was largely driven by the development of new technology, medications that fight infectious diseases, and improved hygiene conditions. But even though we are living longer, we are often suffering from far more chronic diseases—as we learned in previous chapters—as well as disability and age-related decline, which can greatly reduce the quality of those extra years. With longevity, the goal is not just adding years to our lives but promoting health at every age so we can be alert, mobile, and pain- and disease-free for all of our lives.

This is where the WHM as a biohacking module comes in. With the WHM we can biohack our health to live longer and better, naturally and effectively. We do this by tapping into our inner technology, where the self-healing capabilities of our bodies are ignited to continuously restore during the day.

MECHANISMS OF AGING AND LONGEVITY

With each passing year, we become wiser and gain more valuable life experience, and yet, aging can also affect how we look and feel in ways we don't love. At the end of the day, continuing to live means continuing to age. We can't reverse the clock, but we can greatly impact our longevity. In fact, did you know that each of us has two ages? We have a *biological age*—which is the accumulated damage and loss of function in a person's cells over time—and a *chronological age*, which is the actual number of candles on our birthday cake. What's even more interesting is that our biological age can be quite a bit younger or older than our chronological age. How quickly we biologically age is modulated by the interaction between our genes and our environment, and how we respond to stressors in our environment.

In 2009, the Nobel Prize in Physiology or Medicine was given to researchers who uncovered that feelings of stress directly influence the lifespan of humans, by shortening telomeres on DNA. Telomeres are a region of repetitive DNA sequences at the end of a chromosome that protect it from becoming damaged when your cells divide, sort of like the plastic coating at the end of a shoelace, which forms a protective layer and prevents it from fraying. With each cell division, your telomeres become shorter and shorter and thus, there is an interesting link between the length of your telomeres and aging. Research shows that the length of your telomeres is directly linked to your lifespan and quality of life, and that you can increase the length of your telomeres and make them more resilient. Your biological age—which includes how healthy your cells are but also, by extension, how energetic you feel, how your skin glows and hair shines, how quick your cognition is, and how your immune system functions—is something we can influence to a degree.

TELOMERES OVER TIME: People with anxiety, depression, and trauma all have shorter telomeres, but when we work on recovering from these issues, we can make our telomeres more resilient. Research suggests that resilient telomeres can also be passed down to your offspring for three generations if there's no intervention. Cellular aging can start as soon as we become a fertilized egg, as research has shown that if the mother has short telomeres, it directly affects the baby's telomeres. Let it be a reminder that you don't only keep your telomeres healthy and resilient for yourself, you also do it for the next generations.

Just like our risk for mental health issues, we can activate genes associated with longevity and can deactivate genes that increase our risk for age-related decline and disease by exposing ourselves to the right amount and duration of stressors. In fact, experts estimate human lifespan is only 25 percent determined by genetics, and the rest is attributed to how we take care of our bodies. Some experts such as Dr. Kenneth R. Pelletier would argue that it is even closer to 5 percent. Practicing the method gives us natural techniques to optimize our biological age in profound ways to optimize health at every age and stage in our life.

Developing a mindset that faces challenges head-on, as we move through the WHM, can allow stressors to have a rejuvenating effect on our biology instead of a detrimental one. As Dr. Blackburn and Dr. Epel note in their book *The Telomere Effect*, "People who respond to stress by feeling overly threatened have shorter telomeres than people who face stress with a rousing sense of challenge." When we train our minds with the WHM, we can literally rejuvenate our cells. As Dr. Epel stresses: "Don't threaten your telomeres but challenge them." Going beyond your comfort zone is not only beneficial because you overcome your fears and break through limited beliefs, but it also acts like an anti-aging cream.

THE WHM FOR STRESS AND AGING

Prolonged exposure to stress can accelerate aging and cause your telomeres to shorten more quickly, leaving you more vulnerable to age-related symptoms and disease. However, short-term stressors seem to have a protective effect on our biological age, and lead to greater cellular resilience to stress. As we learned in Chapter 2, the WHM is a prime example of this positive type of stress, called hormetic stress. The WHM seems to counteract the impact of stress and aging in a variety of ways.

Cold Shock Proteins

In recent years, the longevity industry has also invested a lot of research into cold shock proteins. When we expose ourselves to low temperatures, such as an ice bath, survival mechanisms are activated to cope with this short-term stress, and one of these is the expression of cold shock proteins in the cells, which have many known revitalizing, rejuvenating, and healing properties, including:

- Encouraging bone growth
- Enhancing wound healing
- Maintaining skeletal muscle
- Activating antioxidant enzymes
- Reducing the loss of muscle mass
- Regulating glucose metabolism and bad cholesterol
- Neuroprotective properties
- Repairing damaged neurons
- Decreasing inflammation
- Stabilizing pro-inflammatory cytokines
- Enhancing autophagy

When we're exposed to the cold, the cells seem to undergo a renewal process, thanks to these cold shock proteins, which also show great promise in the treatment of neurodegenerative diseases such as Alzheimer's. Research shows that the cold can act against neurodegeneration and boost neuroregeneration.

Boosting Blood Flow and Healthy Skin

We already know that the WHM provides a boost for the cardio-vascular system, causing vasoconstriction and vasodilation all over the body and giving the blood vessels a workout. All this increased blood flow and stimulation can be great for skin health and aging. When there is a good blood flow, there is proper delivery of nutrients and oxygen to the cells. When this happens right under the surface of your skin, it ensures the skin is revitalized, leaving it healthy and glowing. Studies have also linked chronic stress to accelerated skin aging through multiple mechanisms, and point to a direct skin-brain connection that is mediated by inflammatory cytokines, hormones, and the HPA axis. Stress, just like too much sun exposure or smoking cigarettes, can damage the skin and make it age prematurely. This makes the Wim Hof Method a great beauty and longevity practice.

The 20-Second Relaxing Ice Facial

By doing this practice, we give ourselves an "ice facial" and a boost of relaxation in just twenty seconds. As mammals, we have an automatic evolutionary response when we submerge our heads in the water, called "the mammalian dive reflex," where we automatically enter a state of calm when our face is underwater. Why? Staying calm offers us the best chance of survival: Mother Nature is truly brilliant! With this practice, we activate this reflex immediately and feel a sense of relaxation as well as receive a great facial since we activate the blood flow and tighten our pores.

How to do it:

Preparation: Fill a bowl of water with ice cubes and stir well for half a minute (making sure the ice melts and the water is very cold).

1. Take a deep breath and immerse your face in the bowl
2. Stay face down under water for about twenty seconds
3. Remove and dry your face

You can do this practice after steaming your face, cleaning your pores, and putting on a face mask, and before putting on your favorite toner, face serum, or day cream. Enjoy the glowing skin and relaxed state!

Increase Insulin Sensitivity

A hallmark of aging is decreasing insulin sensitivity, which regulates our ability to turn blood sugar into energy for the body. When we have poor insulin sensitivity, it means our ability to create energy is compromised, and it leaves us with heightened blood sugar levels, which can lead to prediabetes and eventually Type 2 diabetes, which increases the risk of all kinds of issues and diseases, including blindness, kidney failure, heart attacks, stroke, and lower limb amputation. The numbers of people diagnosed with Type 2 diabetes and prediabetes are on the rise; according to the World Health Organization, the number of people with diabetes rose from 108 million in 1980 to 422 million in 2014.

As we've already learned, cold exposure is a wonderful way to increase our insulin uptake and sensitivity, as it causes our muscles to demand extra energy. Research shows that cold exposure can help people with Type 2 diabetes alleviate their insulin resistance. In one study on overweight and diabetic participants, it was shown that mild cold exposure led to more than 40 percent more insulin sensitivity.

Energy Optimization

Energy is a valuable resource. The WHM can contribute to an increase in cellular energy current in various different ways: by stimulating new mitochondria; increasing ATP production; activating the Cori cycle; increasing red blood cells and creating new blood vessels; boosting noradrenaline, dopamine, and potentially testosterone; getting rid of energy-draining zombie cells and inflammation in the body; and letting us enter a restorative mode. This can explain why most people practicing the WHM mention that it lets them feel more energetic and alive. May the force be with you!

TESTIMONIAL: As a forty-nine-year-old woman and long-time corporate employee, I have faced burnout a few times in my life. One day, deep into my third bout of burnout, which left me sick, tired, and dangerously close to rock bottom, I saw an ad for the Wim Hof Method. I had already tried therapy, self-help books, and powering through my symptoms, so I decided— despite the fact that I was known for absolutely hating the cold—to give this new method a try. I began ending my morning showers with cold water, and it was immediately transformative. A feeling of energy and aliveness replaced my sluggishness, and I kept it up daily because the results were amazing. By the end of the month, I took my first cold bath (46°F) for four minutes. I emerged feeling energized and ecstatic, practically dancing with joy. I also incorporated the Wim Hof breathing technique each morning, finding it calmed me and prepared me for the cold. This health ritual became the cornerstone of my day. The positive effects snowballed—I felt better mentally, my perimenopause symptoms (a significant factor in my burnout) lessened, and my ability to manage stress skyrocketed. Later that year, I became a certified instructor, eager to share the method with others who were struggling the way I had. Today, I'm a certified Wim Hof Method instructor, a life coach, and a trainee in psychotherapy. I help overwhelmed women on the brink of burnout using the Wim Hof Method and other tools.

—Ruth

WEIGHT LOSS AND BROWN FAT ACTIVATION

We can't talk about longevity without talking about weight and metabolism, which can slow down with age and contribute to metabolic disorders. Research shows that spending an hour in 68-degree water increases the metabolic rate by 93 percent, while an hour in 57.2-degree water raises it by an astonishing 350 percent. As we learned in earlier chapters, we ramp up metabolism by producing heat. For example, through shivering, the muscles use glucose. Cold exposure also leads muscles to produce and secrete irisin, a hormone that helps white fat turn into brown fat. Research shows that the presence of brown fat correlates with a healthier metabolism and weight loss, and can be linked to a 50 percent lower risk of Type 2 diabetes and heart disease.

In our community, we have countless stories of practitioners saying they lost weight. Even more fascinating is that the breathwork may actually aid with weight loss, too. How? Research shows that 84 percent of fat loss occurs through breathing, as fat leaves the body in the form of carbon dioxide. For every 10 kilograms of fat metabolized, 8.4 kilograms are exhaled as carbon dioxide, with the remaining 16 percent exiting our body as water. Research also shows that fat cells shrink with deep breathing, helping release carbon dioxide that is "stuck" in the cells. Deep diaphragmatic breathing also massages the organs and boosts metabolism. Ultimately, breathwork may support weight loss in more than one way.

Deep Rest and Sleep

Rest is not a luxury; it's essential for cellular rejuvenation and healthy aging, as well as recovering from the stress of our daily activities. According to the National Institutes of Health, sleep affects every tissue in the body, as well as hormones, the immune system, appetite, mood, breathing, blood pressure, and cardiovascular health.

And yet one in three adults report not getting enough sleep and rest. Lack of sleep is more common in women, with more than half of women getting less than eight hours of sleep (compared to 38 percent of men)—despite studies showing that women actually need more sleep than men. Women are 40 percent more likely to develop insomnia than men, which is often due to anxiety and hormone fluctuations. All this lack of sleep can put us at risk for a myriad of health problems, including heart disease, kidney disease, high blood pressure, diabetes, stroke, obesity, and depression. A recent study on over 172,000 people showed that men and women who get adequate sleep live longer (five years for men and two years for women) than those who don't.

Both the WHM breathing exercises and cold exposure can lead to better sleep. We need our internal temperature to be cooler to fall asleep, but stress tends to activate and heat up our system. Lowering this activation and the body temperature through daily morning cold showers is one way to promote good sleep, as morning cold exposure is closely aligned with our natural cortisol cycle. However, if your nervous system is in overdrive when you get home from work, then a cold shower or ice bath might do the trick in resetting your stress baseline two hours before you go to sleep.

Contrast Protocol: Sleep Like a Baby

Desert ants have an ingenious way to cool off from the smoldering heat. They simply dive deep into the ground, where it's even hotter than on the surface, and then come back up again, feeling a refreshing sense of cool. This is a concept called contrast therapy. The WHM isn't just about getting cold; in fact, contrast with a sauna is actually something we do a lot, especially during our travels, when we train with extreme cold exposure.

When we alternate between cold and heat, we shake up the muscles and the blood vessels and leave ourselves feeling extra relaxed and enjoying a big boost in happy hormones. We often recommend this protocol for promoting high-quality, restorative sleep—you will sleep like a baby!

How to do it:

1. Begin your practice with a cold shower, ice bath, or a dip in natural cold water, if available.
2. While in the cold, practice interoceptive focus by connecting your body and mind. Use your breath to gradually calm yourself. Start by returning your breath to a normal rhythm, inhaling through your nose and exhaling through your mouth. If it feels difficult, try long exhalations or humming. Find comfort in

the discomfort and stay in the cold until you feel mentally and physically adapted.

3. After exiting the cold water, stay focused and mindful of what you're feeling. If you take an ice bath or a cold dip in nature, warm up naturally by practicing the horsestance for a few minutes.

4. Spend about ten minutes in the sauna, staying in until it feels slightly uncomfortable. When it starts to feel challenging, push yourself a little further to enhance the mental and physical benefits. This is when the real exercise begins in the sauna.

5. Alternate between the ice bath and the sauna two to three times. Always end with a cold dip or rinse, even if it's brief, to conclude your practice. This final cold exposure helps your body naturally heat itself up without external sources, effectively "closing the ceremony."

As you can see, the WHM can be an extremely useful biohacking tool to promote longevity and optimal health. It can be used at any age, for any number of common symptoms. If you're using the WHM as a biohacking method, use this Benefit-Based Cold Exposure Guide to fine-tune your practice to your goals.

BENEFIT-BASED COLD EXPOSURE GUIDE

- INCREASE MENTAL AND STRESS RESILIENCE: A two-minute ice bath. It's important to feel uncomfortable and like you would like to get out but use your mind to overcome the challenge and your initial stress response. Overcoming this initial fight-or-flight response teaches us grit and mental resilience.

- MENTAL FOCUS: Noradrenaline flushes through your system in the first twenty seconds at a water temperature between 35.6 and 39.2 degrees. This is the perfect way to get a quick mental boost in little to no time.
- BROWN FAT ACTIVATION: This will occur with any type of cold exposure; just make sure the temperature is 60.8 degrees or below, because that's when brown fat is activated. One study showed that winter swimming for a minimum of eleven minutes a week (and fifty-five minutes of sauna) led to a higher metabolic rate and more brown fat.
- INCREASE INSULIN SENSITIVITY: Mild cold exposure daily. Studies show that ten days of cold exposure (57.2 to 59 degrees) improves insulin sensitivity by 40 percent.
- BOOST HAPPY HORMONES: At least twenty seconds in water between 35.6 and 39.2 degrees will activate noradrenaline and release beta-endorphins in the brain.
- IMPROVE DEPRESSION: Cold showers for two to three minutes daily at 50 to 53.6 degrees. Doing this protocol for a couple of weeks to months relieved symptoms of depression in a study.
- SLEEP: Shower an hour before bed and end it with cold water to lower your core body temperature and relax your mind.
- IMMUNE SYSTEM BOOST: A study in the Netherlands involving three thousand participants found that those who finished their daily shower with a thirty-to-ninety-second blast of cold water reported 29 percent fewer sickness symptoms after just thirty days.
- BUILD MUSCLE: Ice bathing right after a workout is not recommended for muscle building. Instead, take an ice bath before, or wait about four hours before going in.
- INSTANT ENERGY: Any type of cold exposure will do it, including an ice facial, a cold shower, a dip in a cold body of natural water, or an ice bath.

BIOHACK YOUR CYCLE WITH THE WHM

With the WHM we tap into our mind-body connection. Can you listen to the subtle cues of your body? As we always say: feeling is understanding. The reason we say this is that as human beings, especially if you are a techie or a biohacker, we tend to use our minds a lot. But it's essential that we listen to what our bodies have to say, and it's fundamental to the Wim Hof Method. It's possible women could benefit even more than men from using WHM as a biohack practice. Why?

Because we have intricate monthly hormone transitions that affect how we feel and act. Remember, our cold tolerance, breathing rate, carbon dioxide sensitivity, brain chemistry, stress response, metabolism, and thermoregulation all change drastically throughout our cycle. The WHM can help us navigate these changes and fine-tune our wellness practices to optimize our well-being. During our menstrual cycle, we can use the WHM to try to maintain a steadier balance throughout the month, and not only ease but take advantage of the ups and downs we may feel as our hormones shift and change.

Premenstrual and Menstrual Phase: Gloomy Days

Let's start with the part of the cycle that most women find the most difficult: the premenstrual phase and the menstrual phase. If you use a twenty-eight-day cycle as an example, this would be approximately days twenty-five to twenty-eight and the first few days of your period, which are the first days of a new cycle. During this phase there's a decline in progesterone, estrogen, and serotonin, leading to shifts in mood, motivation, and energy. You may feel less stress-resilient and more irritable, and struggle with anxiety, insomnia, and pain. During menstruation, you also shed blood. This loss of blood causes a loss of red blood cells and iron, which can lead to a loss of energy and body heat and interfere with thermoregulation.

Because we are less stress-resilient during this phase, we should be wary of adding fuel to the fire. For many of us, this isn't the best time for extreme cold exposure and instead is the time to focus on breathing and other more comforting practices. If you do want to do cold exposure, we would advise a lighter form, like a cold rinse after your hot shower, or a little hot-cold contrast shower for less than two minutes. Even if you feel good, you're still shedding blood during this time, so we recommend skipping the ice bath until you're at least a few days into your menses.

The WHM Basic Breathing exercise from Chapter 5 (pages 114–15), done while sitting on the couch under a blanket, is often the most beneficial thing to do during this phase. This practice helps ground us and releases emotions that may be stored up, clearing the gloomy skies that are common during this time. Emotional release and regulation are key during this phase and the breathing exercises help us tremendously with this. Many women report that when they can

---

Laura: Although we generally do not recommend extreme cold exposure during menstruation, personally I find that an ice bath helps relieve period pain. The cramping seems to loosen, and the pain starts to subside immediately. I do this while staying fully tuned in to my body and never pushing my limits. The breathing exercises are also a great way to alleviate pain, as they affect our pain perception and have an analgesic effect. By doing a simple three to four rounds of the WHM Basic Breathing exercise, tuning in mentally to the location of the pain, you will feel the cramps subsiding naturally due to the lessening of tension throughout the body. Like anything in the WHM, you can experiment with what feels good to you.

release their pent-up emotions through breathing and regulating their state, they feel much more able to handle the more fragile condition they're in.

The Follicular Phase: The Mood Booster Days

Estrogen starts to rise when your period begins, and by the time your period comes to an end, your confidence, energy, mood, and desire to be outgoing and social are increasing thanks to estrogen's effect. Estrogen is the equivalent of men's testosterone; it's the hormone that gets us ready for action. Estrogen also affects production of serotonin, which is one of the feel-good hormones we learned about in earlier chapters. You might start to feel much more confident and resilient to the cold. Estrogen is a vasodilator, which causes increased blood flow through your whole body, so you feel warmer.

The follicular phase is a great time to ramp up your WHM practices since you'll be feeling more motivated and confident. Both Power Breathing exercises and cold exposure in the form of ice baths and icy dips in natural water are great to do in this phase. Our suggestion for this time: go a little beyond your comfort zone and break through your own limitations!

Ovulation Phase: The Rise-and-Shine Days

Ovulation occurs midway through your cycle, marking the end of the follicular phase as an egg is released from the ovary. This pivotal moment is instigated by a sudden surge in estrogen levels coupled with a rise in luteinizing hormone (LH) and testosterone levels. It's nature's way of preparing your body for potential conception, even if parenthood isn't on your current agenda!

With the peak in estrogen and testosterone, you feel confident, energized, and healthy. You are in a mood to explore new things and challenge yourself. So allow that to be reflected in your WHM practice. If you are up to it, give yourself a challenge and increase your confidence even more.

Some ways to challenge yourself in this phase include:

- Going straight into cold shower, without starting warm
- Increasing your ice bath time from two or three minutes to five minutes
- Doing five rounds of breathing or a round of Power Breathing
- Tracking your retention times. Can you get to three minutes with no breathing during your breathing rounds?

If you can, set a goal during this phase and smash it!

The Luteal Phase: The Introversion Days

After ovulation, the corpus luteum kicks into gear by producing progesterone. This initiates the luteal phase, which lasts from ovulation until menstruation begins. In this phase, progesterone peaks, your energy decreases, your breathing rate increases, and you may feel more introverted. As progesterone increases, you may also feel more relaxed and sleep better because it can stimulate calming neurotransmitters in the brain. The progesterone rise also leads to vasoconstriction and the preservation of heat. Your core body temperature is higher than usual, so other parts of your body, like your hands and feet, can feel colder. You may notice that you dress warmer in this phase than other parts of the cycle and shivering will start earlier than in other phases.

These changes may make you more hesitant to do cold exposure, so a sauna after an ice bath or icy nature swim is a great way to warm up fully and make your practice more comfortable. When you do your breathing, pay attention to the speed and notice if you are falling into that short and shallow breathing pattern that can contribute to stress. When you do the breathing exercises, we recommend sessions that focus on slowing down and deepening your breath to counteract any symptoms you might be experiencing.

Becoming an Icewoman means being in tune with your body and mind and understanding and honoring what it needs at any given time. This can not only make you feel more aligned and relaxed, it can optimize your health at any stage of your life.

BECOMING AN ICEWOMAN

Congratulations! You are entering the final chapter, and now have a wealth of information about not just the Wim Hof Method, but women's health and physiology. You've probably already experimented with a cold shower or two, but if not, don't worry! This is the chapter where we break down exactly how to get started with the three pillars—cold, breath, and mindset—of the WHM.

But before we get to that, it's important to know that once you step into the WHM world, you'll understand that it's actually about more than just these three pillars. In fact, we often talk about three more "hidden WHM pillars." These hidden pillars are intertwined with the WHM experience, each contributing uniquely to our journey of self-discovery, healing, and growth, starting with the nature pillar.

NATURE

We aren't just adjacent to nature, we're part of it! The human body has been created over millions of years of evolution with our environment. Our bodies and minds feel incredibly at ease and at home when we submerge ourselves in nature, with our parasympathetic system instantly activating when we're in water or surrounded by trees. Various cultures have practices that highlight nature's healing powers, such as Japan's "shinrinyoku" (forest bathing), Germany's "waldeinsamkeit" (solitude of the forest), and Finland's "jokamiehenoikeus," which is beautifully translated to "freedom to roam."

Studies have shown that a simple twenty-minute stroll in nature can significantly lower your stress hormone levels and that even a ten-minute walk in nature can meaningfully reduce burnout. Others show that a day trip to the forest reduces cortisol and adrenaline for up to seven days and that two nights in nature proved 50 percent more effective in reducing burnout than mindfulness. Sadly, 25 percent of Americans spend their whole days indoors with less than an hour of sun or fresh air exposure. Research is very clear that nature sounds, nature environments, and even environments that mimic nature have a positive and healing effect on our physical and mental health.

Connecting with the natural world has always been an intrinsic part of the WHM, which is why we often hold our retreats surrounded by nature. Wim didn't have an ice bath in the early days; the WHM was born in lakes and oceans and streams. As kids, winter was our favorite season, and we would watch our dad go into the frozen lake in the park next to our house every single day or spend time in the Spanish Pyrenees, a mountain range close to the town where our mother was raised. Our dad even bought a small house in Poland, just because it was around the corner from an amazing waterfall. Funny enough, our dad now has a pool, but he only uses it during winter. He prefers the lake, where he can get in tune with his natural surroundings. This is also why we recommend doing your WHM practice while surrounded by nature whenever possible. Being in nature for the breathing exercises and cold exposure maximizes their benefits, and brings you to an even deeper feeling of connection and calm. In nature, we clear our minds and recharge our batteries.

THE EXCHANGE OF LIFE FORCE: When we submerge ourselves in the natural world, we also form a perfect symbiosis with nature where we exchange our life force with our surroundings. Just like your lungs, a tree consists of a large trunk that leads to thousands of smaller branches. Lungs look like an upside-down tree, with branches moving into millions of intricate passages. Trees absorb carbon dioxide from the air, which they assimilate with water to produce glucose, and in turn, they release oxygen into the atmosphere. We operate in the opposite manner. We inhale oxygen, which we combine with glucose to generate energy, releasing carbon dioxide and water as a by-product into the environment. In other words, the stuff we breathe out is what trees breathe in, and the stuff trees breathe out, we breathe in! Trees and humans need each other.

COMMUNITY

Anyone who experienced COVID-19 times can attest to the fact that we are social beings. And as women, our deep urge to "tend and befriend" is a fundamental survival mechanism. Having people around us who we trust and connect with makes us feel safe, especially when we experience stressful situations. The mere presence of others can bring out the best in us! Women are often the backbone and social structure of communities, building and maintaining important relationships within and between groups. Women thrive when they feel part of a community.

All of this is why we formed the Icewomen Community, and why connection-building is such a big aspect of our WHM retreats and travels. The act of doing the ice bath for the first time as an individual is one thing. But doing it together? That creates lifelong bonds.

Similarly, doing group breathing sessions—where we get to release trauma, be vulnerable, and cry in a safe space with others—can create an even more powerful, lasting impact. Breaking down in a group of mostly strangers can feel intimidating, but when you allow others to witness your emotions and they acknowledge them with love and compassion, it can lead to profound breakthroughs. When we are fully accepted by others in our most true and authentic form, we are often hit with the realization that we are enough, and we are perfect just the way we are. This happens quickly in the context of others, who act as mirrors to our souls and help us release more oxytocin, which works to counterbalance the effect of cortisol and promotes feelings of love, safety, and relaxation.

The Icewomen Community was born just before COVID times, but greatly expanded during the pandemic, and acts as a way for women to come together to dip and make beautiful connections. Many women credit the community for their introduction into the WHM. This Wim Hof Method community has helped thousands of women push through limiting beliefs, transform their mindset, and of course, make new friendships that will last a lifetime!

PLAY

If there is one thing that's evident on our WHM retreats, it's that we have fun! We cry, we dance, we laugh, we make jokes, and we don't take anything too seriously. We can have fun even when we're in the ice bath, when we're releasing emotions or facing a challenge. By approaching difficulties in a playful manner, we allow ourselves to learn fast and truly understand the depth of the WHM. Scientists seem to agree that play enables us to learn quicker, showing that neurological changes are made easier when we have fun.

When we have fun, we can also allow our creativity to flourish.

Many professional musicians and artists have found new inspiration by practicing the WHM.

During our retreats you will often hear about the "no program program," which means we have a loose schedule, but anything can change at any moment. For very structured people who are used to knowing exactly what is going to happen and when, our retreats can be an exercise in letting go. We encourage you to take this approach with your own practice, even if you're not attending a retreat with a WHM practitioner. Allow yourself to lean into the fun and playfulness of it all. Not being too stringent with your practice can help you connect your body and mind, and be much more in the moment—because that is what play is all about! No need to think about what is next, just being in the here and now. As we always say: "Trust the process." Play is the ultimate exercise in letting go.

Now that you know the hidden pillars of the Wim Hof Method, it's time to start your practice.

BECOMING AN ICEWOMAN: HOW TO START

As you've learned, the Wim Hof Method isn't one single protocol. In fact, it includes a variety of protocols that you can mix and match in your personal practice. In scientific research of the WHM, though, our science liaison tailors the methodology precisely according to the specific aim with the utmost care.

The versatility of the method creates a wonderful opportunity to tailor the method to specific health goals or issues, or simply adapt it to what your body and mind need on any day as you hone your mind-body connection. We encourage you to find what works best for you. The ideal approach is to choose a cold practice that you can consistently maintain and make your own.

That said, we know that for absolute beginners, too many choices can feel overwhelming. That's why we created this easy 30-Day Icewoman Challenge, specifically for all the women reading this book—to use as a starting point on which you can slowly build. It will help you ease into the fundamentals of the WHM in a structured way, and also help you establish a WHM practice that actually becomes a habit, so you can get the long-term benefits. Two of the fundamental protocols you'll be doing are WHM Basic Breathing (pages 114–15) and WHM Power Breathing (pages 117–18).

This thirty-day guide will ease you into our breathing, cold exposure, and mindset exercises to help you fully integrate the Wim Hof Method into your life. Each day, you'll progressively build your resilience, both physically and mentally, and learn to integrate the method into your life in a meaningful way. The real practice starts after the thirty days. Of course, listen to your body and feel free to skip a day here and there, but the rule is: don't skip more than one day!

We recommend using the QR code to access a digital version of the 30-Day Icewoman Challenge and printing the challenge out to hang it somewhere prominent, like on your fridge or bathroom door, so you can cross off each day you complete. Or download the Wim Hof Method app and keep track there. We highly recommend doing the Icewoman Challenge with a buddy to keep it playful and build more connection through the experience. And don't forget to tag #Icewoman30days on social media to motivate other women to join the movement!

Week 1: The Fundamentals

Days 1–3: Introducing Breathing, Cold Exposure, and Mindset

The first three days are all about the fundamentals. Before you start, reflect on what you want to achieve during the challenge, and write your thoughts down on paper. Write down possible obstacles to finishing this challenge and how you plan to overcome them.

- BREATHWORK: Begin each morning before breakfast and coffee with three rounds of WHM Basic Breathing.
- COLD EXPOSURE: Start with a ten-second cold shower at the end of your regular warm shower on day one and then increase to fifteen seconds and twenty seconds on days two and three.
- MINDSET: Start your breathing practices with a strong intention. Think about why you wanted to start this thirty-day challenge and set an intention to finish the full thirty days. Prepare mentally and physically by doing the "Setting an Intention" exercise on page 136. Before you start your first cold shower, relax your shoulders and tell yourself, "I can do this."

Days 4–7: Building Consistency

You've been at it for three days already! Your cold showers may already feel more natural than on day one. Let's see if we can further the practice by starting to "welcome" the cold. This means relaxing into the cold and finding calm despite the stress of the cold. *Be strong through discomfort and stay in control of your mind.*

- BREATHWORK: Continue with three rounds of WHM Basic Breathing and pay close attention to how your body responds. Tingling sensations, buzzing, strong emotions, it's all okay.
- COLD EXPOSURE: Increase your cold shower time to twenty-five seconds on day four, thirty seconds on day five,

thirty-five seconds on day six, and forty seconds on day seven. Focus on relaxing into the cold.

- MINDSET: The moment before you enter the cold, set your intention. Say to yourself, "I am in control." As you try to relax into the cold, get ready for thoughts and feelings to arise. Oftentimes, these thoughts are your inner saboteur coming up to tell you to skip a day of cold practice, or just rinse for a few seconds instead of the full twenty-five or forty. Focus on taking the reins over your inner saboteur and your body and mind. You can say out loud: "I am in control."

Week 2: Deepen Your Practice

Days 8–10: Enhancing Breathing and Cold Tolerance

As you deepen your practice, focus on starting each day with gratitude and a can-do mindset. Tackle the shower and breathwork like you're tackling the day, with compassion and care for yourself.

- BREATHWORK: Increase to four rounds of WHM Basic Breathing if it feels comfortable.
- COLD EXPOSURE: Extend your cold showers to forty-five seconds on day eight, fifty seconds on day nine, and fifty-five seconds on day ten. If you are up to doing more, that's also great. Keep it at a maximum of two minutes, though.
- MINDSET: Start each breathing session by setting an intention and dedicate yourself consciously to your practice. Start your cold exposure with a can-do mindset. Tackle the shower like you'd want to tackle the day, with compassion and care for yourself, while accepting discomfort. Write down three things you're grateful for each morning after your breathwork practice.

Days 11–14: Introducing Advanced Breathing and Mental Resilience

After your usual breathing sessions, give yourself some time to stay in a meditative state and observe the messages you receive from your body and mind. In a state of relaxation, we often get clarity about our goals, our needs, and any decisions we need to make. Just give yourself space and time to feel and let the thoughts enter your consciousness freely.

Set a personal goal for the end of the thirty days.

- BREATHWORK: Introduce WHM Power Breathing on day eleven. If possible, implement it on a weekend day, and do this only if you're comfortable with the Basic Breathing. The Power Breathing goes beyond typical breathwork, so you really must feel ready for it.
- COLD EXPOSURE: Increase your cold shower times to one minute on day eleven, one minute and fifteen seconds on day twelve, one minute and thirty seconds on day thirteen, and one minute and forty-five seconds on day fourteen.
- MINDSET: Set a strong intention for your Power Breathing and give it your all. Reflect on your progress. What challenges have you faced, and how have you overcome them? For your usual breathing sessions, give yourself some time after to stay in the meditative state. What kind of messages are you receiving? In this state of relaxation, we often gain clarity about our goals, our needs, and what directions to take.

Week 3: Go Beyond Your Comfort Zone

Days 15–17: Try Your First Ice Bath

It's time to try your first ice bath! As you do your practice, become aware of your inner voice. Is what it's telling you true? Become aware of any conditioned thoughts or feelings. Then flip the script and be as compassionate as you can toward yourself. Learn to listen to this voice with a smile and then change the narrative by instead talking to yourself like you would soothe or encourage your best friend.

- BREATHWORK: Stick with three or four rounds of WHM Basic Breathing and include one Power Breathing session.
- COLD EXPOSURE: It's time to try your first ice bath! On one of the days, try to submerge in the ice bath for two minutes at 32 to 39.2 degrees. On the other days, do a two-minute cold shower.
- MINDSET: Each day after your breathing exercises, take ten minutes to stay still and meditate. Try leaning into the power of visualization: imagine living your perfect day, achieving your ideal self, and crushing your goals for the week. Remember, visualization is simply a mental rehearsal for the real thing and can greatly increase your chances of success! Before each cold exposure, talk to yourself as you would to a close friend. Focus on your resilience and strength. Mirror yourself and just observe whatever thoughts come up. What is the voice in your head trying to tell you? It often speaks to your conditioned response toward discomfort in life. Learn to listen to it with a smile.

Days 18–22: Connect with Your Body and Emotions

More isn't always better. While we've worked to slowly increase your cold exposure time to increase your cold tolerance, now is the time to reflect on what feels best to you. This means listening to your body and focusing on the amount of time that feels like just enough. Focus on challenging yourself in a way that feels healthy and encouraging, versus overly harsh or punishing.

- BREATHWORK: Complete anywhere between one round and five rounds of WHM Basic Breathing. If you're feeling up to it, do a Power Breathing exercise on day twenty-one.
- COLD EXPOSURE: On all but one of the days, do a cold shower for the amount of time that feels right to you, anywhere from fifteen seconds to two minutes. On the last day, try to find a place to do an ice bath surrounded by nature, or dip in natural water. If that's not possible, stick with a cold shower.
- MINDSET: Before doing your breathing exercise each day, do the Interoception of the Heartbeat (page 137) to slow down and help connect your mind and body. During your Power Breathing session, connect with your emotions. Accept the emotions that arise. If you want, you might connect with your inner child. Talking to your inner child is a tremendous and powerful way to release old trauma. Accept it and let it go.

Week 4: Master and Manifest

Days 23–25: Refining Your Practice

As you do your practices this week, especially the two-to-three-minute ice bath challenge, try to connect with your inner child. Imagine yourself as a kid and tell yourself things you wish you'd heard then. It could be words of support, validation, or kindness. This is a tremendous and powerful way to release stored-up emotions, pain, or trauma. Accept anything that comes up and allow it to flow out of you.

- BREATHWORK: Return to three to four rounds of WHM Basic Breathing every day. You can also include Power Breathing every other day, deciding based on how you feel which days to push yourself and which days you need more rest. Don't hold back this week, it is the last phase!

- COLD EXPOSURE: Challenge yourself with a two-to-three-minute ice bath on day twenty-three. Stick with one-to-two-minute cold showers on the other days.
- MINDSET: Reflect on your journey so far and write down your responses to the following questions: What have you learned about yourself? How has your mindset shifted? Have you identified any limiting beliefs, and if yes, what are they? What would happen if you let those beliefs go? Before your breath practice, set an intention to release these limiting beliefs.

Days 26–29: Aligning with Your Goals

On these final days of the challenge, try to draw a connection between facing this challenge and the challenges in your life. Ask yourself: What is it you most want in life? What would make you your healthiest, happiest, and truest self?

- BREATHWORK: On one of the days, consider doing five rounds of WHM Basic Breathing if you feel comfortable. Otherwise, continue with three to four rounds of WHM Basic Breathing.
- COLD EXPOSURE: Aim for a nature dip with somebody. Cold showers remain daily, one to two minutes. Focus on mental clarity and overcoming the body's initial resistance.
- MINDSET: After your breathing practice, take ten to fifteen minutes to be still and think about your life goals. What is it that you most want in life? Think about it like you are limitless. During your cold exposure, continue your thoughts of being limitless. Imagine yourself as someone who can do whatever she sets her mind to. Repeat your own "unlimited" mantra: "I can do whatever I want. I am capable of anything I set my mind to. I am unstoppable."

Day 30: Becoming an Invincible Icewoman

You faced the ice bath with strength, confidence, and kindness toward yourself. Can you face the challenges in your real life with the same mindset? During your cold exposure, imagine yourself as an invincible being who can do anything she sets her mind to. Create your own Invincible Icewoman mantra—like "Anything I wish for manifests itself with ease and grace"—and repeat it while you are in the cold.

- BREATHWORK: Do a final session with five rounds of WHM Basic Breathing and two rounds of Power Breathing.
- COLD EXPOSURE: End the challenge with a three-to-five-minute ice bath or nature dip if available.
- MINDSET: Reflect on the entire thirty days. Write down how you feel, what you've learned, and how you've grown. Set intentions for maintaining this practice in your life moving forward. During your breath practice, give yourself a mental high five. Remind yourself you are perfect just the way you are.

Congratulations! You've completed the 30-Day Icewoman Challenge. You've not only enhanced your physical resilience, but you've also cultivated a stronger, more resilient mindset.

If we've learned anything in our years of teaching the WHM, it's that after just thirty days of practice, you'll become calmer, more resilient, and more energetic and confident. And this won't benefit only you. When we're able to be our best selves, it benefits later generations, too.

COOL KIDS

We don't only become Icewomen for ourselves, we do it for our children! Our stress can have a physiological effect on our children's nervous system, something called "stress contagion." In one study, twelve-to-fourteen-month-old infants were placed on the laps of mothers who were stressed, and the babies showed increased sympathetic activity. The balance we reach when doing the method will no doubt benefit the next generation. But can our kids do the WHM with us?

We get this question frequently in our trainings, and there is a historical basis for possible cold exposure benefits for kids. In Siberia and Scandinavia, babies are often wrapped up in blankets and left to nap outside. In Russia and Scandinavia, children are sometimes brought outside to play in the snow barefoot, dunked in a bucket of ice water, or even submerged in an ice hole during Orthodox Christian Epiphany. Similarly, Native American tribes are said to have given their babies a snow bath, a tradition among some tribes that still lives on today. In most of these cases, cold exposure is thought to help the child build up their immunity!

Just a few years ago, a day care in the Netherlands gave a group of three-year-olds the option to briefly walk in the snow in their bare feet. The activity sparked a lot of controversy among parents—some were outraged, going so far as to label it child abuse—and many newspapers and talk shows covered the conflict. Naturally, the WHM organization was asked to weigh in on the matter, and our comments stressed that such intense reactions from parents often stem from the ingrained belief that cold is inherently harmful. But cold exposure, when brief and controlled, can be highly beneficial for children. Just a few moments of exposure can activate their nervous system, followed by a period of rest that improves their mood and overall well-being. Remember, children also still have their brown fat. Of course, with the Iceman as our father, we had a lot of experience with the cold as kids, but our father never forced us and instead gave us the space to decide for ourselves how much of the cold we wanted to experiment with. This approach is always what we tell parents to follow. The goal is to be the example as a parent and welcome them into the process if they show interest, but always let your kid decide for themselves.

When it comes to the breathing exercises, our children may already have a leg up on us! Kids and babies breathe naturally into their bellies. It's with age and the stress that comes with it that these patterns can change into less healthy ones. In Dutch we have a saying, "Jong geleerd, is oud gedaan," which means "Learned young, is done old."

Isabelle: I firmly believe that by teaching the younger generation the importance of healthy breathing habits, we are planting seeds that will nurture their well-being. When we practice conscious breathing with a focus on breathing correctly for a few minutes a day with our children, this will be stored up in our unconscious and conscious as something we always carry and can put our focus on whenever we want. Proactively engaging with cold exposure can help to regulate intense emotion in the face of adversity; after all, the cold is like an emotion!

However, when it comes to the WHM breathing exercises, it's crucial that they are adapted to suit the developmental stage of the child. For children under eight, we recommend simply bringing attention to the breath or incorporating play by blowing up a balloon together. For children over eight, we suggest this adaptation of the WHM Basic Breathing.

Protocol: The WHM Cool Kids Breathing Exercise

1. **GET COMFORTABLE:** Sit or lie down comfortably, or whichever way is most comfortable for you.
2. **BREATHE CONSCIOUSLY:** Become aware of your breath, follow it, and try to fully connect with it. If a thought arises, welcome it and let it go by refocusing on the breath.
3. **TWENTY DEEP BREATHS:** You can close your eyes if you want to. Inhale deeply through the nose and exhale unforced through the mouth. Fully inhale into the belly, then the chest, and then let go unforced. Focus on a long exhale. Do this twenty times.
4. **THE HOLD:** After the twenty deep breaths, draw the breath in once more and fill the lungs to maximum capacity without forcing it. Then let the air out and hold for a maximum of twenty seconds.
5. **RECOVERY BREATH:** After twenty seconds, draw one breath in. Feel your belly and chest expanding, and when you are at full capacity, hold your breath for around five seconds. Then let go. This is one round. This breathing exercise can be repeated for two to three rounds, one after another.

After the breathing sessions, enjoy the feeling and talk together about how your body and mind feel before and after the breathing.

Protocol: Breathe Like a Musician

This breathing exercise is perfect if your child is facing an emotional situation and needs a quick way to calm down. It's a simple and effective way to help your child get a handle on their heart rate and intense emotions.

1. Take a deep breath through the nose.
2. Sing do-re-mi-fa-so-la-ti-do until you have fully exhaled all the air.
3. Repeat this a few times, or until they start to calm down.

The WHM offers you and your kids a great way to bond, play, challenge yourselves, and connect with nature. By doing it as a family, you are helping establish a lifestyle. Because if you're going to reap long-term benefits from the WHM, commitment is *key*.

HOW TO MAKE THE WHM A LASTING PRACTICE

The brain's remarkable plasticity means that there are endless opportunities to change and form new habits. And yet creating lasting change isn't as simple as a single WHM session. Scientific research suggests embedding new habits into our daily lives requires around sixty-six days of consistent practice. Research shows that these days aren't without their challenges; the first twenty-two days can be particularly tough as we cling to familiar comforts, like our beloved warm showers in the case of the WHM. The following twenty-two days can be a whirlwind of adaptation, as we start to recognize the possible benefits of the new habit. With the WHM, you may find that you start to appreciate certain aspects of the cold and breathing, and that your mindset is changing for the better. Finally, in the last stretch of twenty-two days, we find ourselves embracing and enjoying our newfound habits. At the end of this journey, the new habit becomes seamlessly woven into our daily routines.

That said, many of us don't reach the end of this journey. Initially, enthusiasm runs high, but as time passes, the reality of how much work this change will require sets in. Research indicates that only a fraction of people will persist with their goals three weeks later, and even fewer will maintain them after two months. After all, all kinds of domestic and professional things clutter our days, fill our agendas, and hinder our focus. Often, the issue lies not in lack of intention but in the lack of an effective strategy and understanding of our own behaviors and psychology. Whether it's adopting the WHM or pursuing any other behavioral change, initial motivation can only carry us so far. Studies, such as a systematic review encompassing 422 research papers, reveal that mere intentions account for just 28 percent of our actual behaviors. While a strong intention serves as a solid foundation, sustainable change demands more. As you start your regular WHM practice, lean on these strategies and techniques to create sustainable change.

1. **Define your why**

   There are various motivations for practicing the WHM. Are you aiming to mitigate stress, enhance your mood, boost overall well-being, increase cold tolerance, or address specific health concerns? It's crucial to have a clear "why" when you are establishing this new practice. This clarity will serve as a cornerstone for maintaining consistency in your practice.

2. **Create if-then plans**

   Isabelle here! Understanding what causes effective habit change is one of my passions, so much so that I got a master's degree in health psychology. This education involved a lot of learning about the science behind behavioral change and how to form lasting habits. I also worked for the health department, where I led initiatives to create healthy behavioral change in communities. After all this experience in this field, I can tell you one of the most interesting and effective strategies in behavioral change is implementation intention. An implementation intention is a strategy that helps us create a regular WHM practice without relying on willpower alone. By formulating a clear plan, we increase the likelihood of reaching a behavior goal and creating a useful habit. Oftentimes, we have no issue in formulating a goal, but following up on the steps to reach the goal can be a bit more challenging. By specifying why, when, where, and how, we can transform a goal into a successful long-term lifestyle change.

Examples of if-then plans:

- If I wake up in the morning, then I start doing three rounds of WHM breathing.
- If I take a shower, then I start my shower warm and then finish it with two minutes cold.
- If I arrive home after a busy day, I will do at least three rounds of WHM breathing right away to transition into the evening.
- If I feel angry or sad or overwhelmed by my emotions, instead of reacting I will do the WHM Basic Breathing exercise.

3. **Obstacles**

Obstacles will no doubt appear on your path, so it's better to be prepared! Reflect on what might get in the way of a regular WHM and what you can do to overcome them.

- What could make practicing the WHM consistently difficult for you?
- What are solutions to overcome these difficulties?

4. **Set reminders**

One effective way to change behavior is to use reminders to help us with our behavioral goals. For example, you can hang a Post-it note in an obvious place like your bathroom mirror, or wear a bracelet that reminds you of your goal. When you see the reminder, your intention or goal will be activated and reinforced.

5. **Create accountability and community**

Forming community around a new habit increases the chance that the habit will last; at the end of the day, we are all social animals. Luckily, when it comes to the WHM, there are endless opportunities to connect with other "Hoffers." For example, you could:

- Join one of the Icewomen communities or create your own!
- Visit Hoffers abroad and connect with people in the local area at their favorite place to practice.
- Connect with the WHM community through the internet.
- Go on a WHM retreat!

6. **Reward yourself**

Remember when you were little, and you got a sticker when you did your homework? A reward felt great then, and it'll feel great as an adult, too. As adults, rewards can take many forms, but one we recommend is simply giving yourself a lot of credit for what you accomplished. Congratulating and complimenting ourselves acts as a boost of magical energy pushing us further in the direction we want to go. Give yourself credit if you did a certain behavior, especially when it was hard. This will motivate you to do it again next time.

A FINAL MESSAGE TO OUR NEWEST ICEWOMEN

We have taught the Wim Hof Method to thousands of women all over the world, forming deep connections along the way. We have offered words of comfort and encouragement during their first ice bath, shared uncontrollable laughter during our women-only retreats, and held space as many emotions and painful memories have been released. We have learned so much about the lives of so many women and found that if there is one experience that seems to unite us all, it's a sinking feeling that we are not good enough. For some, it's a subtle occasional pang of doubt; for others, it's an overwhelming and all-encompassing belief that shapes how they move through life. Practicing the Wim Hof Method helps dissolve this ever-present fear, allowing us to finally embrace the truth: we are enough, exactly as we are, right now.

The world looks so much brighter and more colorful after even just one good WHM session. We've witnessed countless women grow more confident and fearless, taking on challenges they once hesitated to face. Together, we break through the conditioning, limiting beliefs, and fears that have held us back, and begin to see life through a lens of growth. With this new perspective, challenges become opportunities, and we step into a mindset that empowers us to break free from old patterns and create a new reality grounded in trust and self-belief.

When we do the WHM breathing and cold exposure, there is nowhere to hide. The layers that formed around you throughout the years will fade away, and you will connect deeply to your vulnerable and powerful self. You reconnect with your inner voice. What are your true feelings? What do you wish for? What do you really need? What do you have to say? As unnecessary baggage dissolves, you journey forward in your most authentic form, just the way you were always meant to be.

ACKNOWLEDGMENTS

We would like to express our deepest gratitude to everyone who contributed to making this book a reality.

We want to honor and thank our parents, whose love, resilience, and influence have been central to this journey. To our father, who has devoted his life to a mission of helping others become happy, strong, and healthy: your dedication and persistence has inspired not just this book but an entire movement. To our mother, whose profound sacrifices and enduring spirit continue to guide us: your passing was the catalyst for a mission that became a family endeavor to heal and inspire the world.

To our brother Enahm Hof, who created a platform so that these powerful techniques could become accessible to the world, and to our brother Michael Hof, whose steady contributions at the roots have been essential for the method.

To our publisher, Karen, and our editors, Gretchen and Kirby: your invaluable guidance and dedication played a pivotal role in shaping this book into its final form.

To our trusted liaison Jaidree, who has been our guide, adviser, and anchor. Jaidree was instrumental in transforming the initial vision of this book into reality. We are incredibly fortunate to have had her by our side every step of the way.

We are immensely grateful to all Wim Hof Method instructors, especially the remarkable women in this field, and the incredible

Icewomen Community leaders and Hoffers: your contributions, participation, and passion have enriched this work in countless ways. And a big heads-up to the women who are sharing their personal stories with the WHM for this book: your testimonial will motivate other women to step into this practice to alleviate certain health issues even more!

To all the experts who generously shared their time and insights with us—your contributions have been invaluable, and we are honored to have had the privilege of learning and reflecting from and with you: Prof. Dr. Elissa Epel; Prof. Dr. Wouter van Marken Lichtenbelt; Prof. Dr. Hemmo Drexhage; Prof. Dr. Max Nieuwdorp; Peter M. Litchfield; Prof. Henk Jan den Boele, MD; Andrew Weil, MD; Prof. Matthias Wittfoth; and hormonal expert Ralph Moorman.

I, Isabelle, wish to express my heartfelt thanks to my partner, Oren Gatigno, for your unwavering support as we balanced the demands of writing this book with raising a (newborn) baby.

Finally, to everyone who supported us along the way: thank you for believing in this vision and helping bring it to life. This book is as much yours as it is ours.

NOTES

CHAPTER 1: THE WIM HOF METHOD

3   Dr. Kamler's team observed: Ken Kamler, MD, and Granis Stewart, RN, Letter to WHM Services Unipessoal LDA - Innerfire BV, September 17, 2009, https://media-cdn.wimhofmethod.com/uploads/kcfinder/files/WHM _DataInfo%20Kamler.pdf.

4   the 2012 study: Matthijs Kox, PhD, et al., "The Influence of Concentration/ Meditation on Autonomic Nervous System Activity and the Innate Immune Response: A Case Study," *Psychosomatic Medicine* 74, no. 5 (2012): 489–94, 10.1097/PSY.0b013e3182583c6d.

6   The results of this study: Matthijs Kox, PhD, et al., "Voluntary Activation of the Sympathetic Nervous System and Attenuation of the Innate Immune Response in Humans," *Proceedings of the National Academy of Sciences* 111, no. 20 (2014): 7379–84, doi:10.1073/pnas.1322174111.

7   including women in 2009: Elizabeth Cooney, "Females Still Routinely Left Out of Biomedical Research—and in Analyses," STAT, June 9, 2020, https://www.statnews.com/2020/06/09/females-are-still-routinely-left -out-of-biomedical-research-and-ignored-in-analyses-of-data/.

7   twice the rate of men: Irving Zucker and Brian J. Prendergast, "Sex Differences in Pharmacokinetics Predict Adverse Drug Reactions in Women," *Biology of Sex Differences* 11, no. 1 (June 5, 2020), https://doi.org/10.1186 /s13293-020-00308-5.

7   to 49 percent in 2019: Cooney, "Females Still Routinely Left Out of Biomedical Research—and in Analyses."

7   preliminary results showed: Dr. Elizabeth Blackburn and Dr. Elissa Epel, *The Telomere Effect: A Revolutionary Approach to Living Younger, Healthier, Longer* (New York: Grand Central Publishing, 2017).

12   pillars is the strongest: Jelle Zwaag, Rick Naaktgeboren, Antonius E. van Herwaarden, Peter Pickkers, and Matthijs Kox, "The Effects of Cold Exposure Training and a Breathing Exercise on the Inflammatory Response in Humans: A Pilot Study," *Psychosomatic Medicine* 84, no. 4 (February 23, 2022): 457–67, https://doi.org/10.1097/psy.0000000000001065.

CHAPTER 2: WOMEN AND THE STRESS OF A MAN'S WORLD

16   this homeostatic balance: Neil Schneiderman, Gail Ironson, and Scott D. Siegel, "Stress and Health: Psychological, Behavioral, and Biological Determinants," *Annual Review of Clinical Psychology* 1, no. 1 (April 1, 2005): 607–28, https://doi.org/10.1146/annurev.clinpsy.1.102803.144141.

17   bits per second: Ap Dijksterhuis, *The Smart Unconscious: Thinking with and Beyond Our Brain* (Amsterdam: Amsterdam University Press, 2007).

17   stability through change: Douglas S. Ramsay and Stephen C. Woods, "Clarifying the Roles of Homeostasis and Allostasis in Physiological Regulation," *Psychological Review* 121, no. 2 (2014): 225–47, https://doi.org/10.1037/a0035942.

20   and digestion: Harvard Health, "Understanding the Stress Response," June 15, 2011, https://www.health.harvard.edu/staying-healthy/understanding-the-stress-response.

21   main contributing factor: Mohd Razali Salleh, "Life Event, Stress and Illness," *Malaysian Journal of Medical Sciences: MJMS* 15, no. 4 (2008): 9–18.

22   to potential threats: Tatia M. C. Lee, Chetwyn C. H. Chan, Ada W. S. Leung, Peter T. Fox, and Jia-Hong Gao, "Sex-Related Differences in Neural Activity During Risk Taking: An fMRI Study," *Cerebral Cortex* 19, no. 6 (June 2009): 1303–12, https://doi.org/10.1093/cercor/bhn172.

23   *twice as likely*: Olivia Remes, Carol Brayne, Rianne van der Linde, and Louise Lafortune, "A Systematic Review of Reviews on the Prevalence of Anxiety Disorders in Adult Populations," *Brain and Behavior* 6, no. 7 (June 5, 2016), https://doi.org/10.1002/brb3.497.

23   in 2000 by Shelley Taylor: Shelley E. Taylor, "Tend and Befriend Theory," in *Handbook of Theories of Social Psychology*, vol. 1 (London: SAGE Publications, 2012), 32–49, http://dx.doi.org/10.4135/9781446249215.n3.

23   response was first named: Theodore M. Brown and Elizabeth Fee, "Walter Bradford Cannon," *American Journal of Public Health* 92, no. 10 (October 2002): 1594–95, https://doi.org/10.2105/ajph.92.10.1594.

24   active in female brains: (Iris Else Clara) Sommer, "The Female Brain," University of Groningen research portal, accessed October 16, 2024, https://research.rug.nl/en/publications/het-vrouwenbrein.

24   include the amygdala: Elizabeth V. Goldfarb, Dongju Seo, and Rajita Sinha, "Sex Differences in Neural Stress Responses and Correlation with Subjective Stress and Stress Regulation," *Neurobiology of Stress* 11 (November 2019): 100177, https://doi.org/10.1016/j.ynstr.2019.100177.

25   nonpromotable tasks: Linda Babcock, Maria P. Recalde, Lise Vesterlund, and Laurie Weingart, "Gender Differences in Accepting and Receiving Requests for Tasks with Low Promotability," *American Economic Review* 107, no. 3 (March 1, 2017): 714–47, https://doi.org/10.1257/aer.20141734.

25   heightened risk of burnout: Lydia Saad, Sangeeta Agrawal, and Ben Wigert, "Gender Gap in Worker Burnout Widened amid the Pandemic," Gallup, December 27, 2021, https://www.gallup.com/workplace/358349/gender-gap-worker-burnout-widened-amid-pandemic.aspx.

25   more sleep than men: Sarah A. Burgard and Jennifer A. Ailshire, "Gender and Time for Sleep Among U.S. Adults," *American Sociological Review* 78, no. 1 (January 30, 2013): 51–69, https://doi.org/10.1177/0003122412472048.

25   experience insomnia: Monica P. Mallampalli and Christine L. Carter, "Exploring Sex and Gender Differences in Sleep Health: A Society for Women's Health Research Report," *Journal of Women's Health* 23, no. 7 (July 2014): 553–62, https://doi.org/10.1089/jwh.2014.4816.

25   736 million women: UN Women – Headquarters, "Facts and Figures: Ending Violence Against Women," accessed October 16, 2024, https://www.unwomen.org/en/what-we-do/ending-violence-against-women/facts-and-figures.

26   connections within the amygdala: B. S. McEwen, C. Nasca, and J. D. Gray, "Stress Effects on Neuronal Structure: Hippocampus, Amygdala, and Prefrontal Cortex," *Neuropsychopharmacology: Official Publication of the American College of Neuropsychopharmacology* 41, no. 1 (2016): 3–23, https://doi.org/10.1038/npp.2015.171.

26   robust neuroendocrine response: Mario G. Oyola and Robert J. Handa, "Hypothalamic-Pituitary-Adrenal and Hypothalamic-Pituitary-Gonadal Axes: Sex Differences in Regulation of Stress Responsivity," *Stress* 20, no. 5 (September 2017): 476–94, https://doi.org/10.1080/10253890.2017.1369523.

28   members of an Antarctic expedition: Tereza Petraskova Touskova, Petr Bob, Zdenek Bares, Zdislava Vanickova, Daniel Nyvlt, and Jiri Raboch, "A Novel Wim Hof Psychophysiological Training Program to Reduce Stress Responses During an Antarctic Expedition," *Journal of International Medical Research* 50, no. 4 (April 2022): 3000605221089883, https://doi.org/10.1177/03000605221089883.

29   for just six weeks: Otto Muzik, Timothy Mann, John Kopchick, Asadur Chowdury, Mario Yacou, Jamie Vadgama, Daniel Bonello, and Vaibhav A. Diwadkar, "The Impact of a Focused Behavioral Intervention on Brain Cannabinoid Signaling and Interoceptive Function: Implications for Mood and Anxiety," *Brain Behavior and Immunity Integrative* 5 (January 2024): 100035, https://doi.org/10.1016/j.bbii.2023.100035.

29   results were most pronounced: Cristopher Siegfried Kopplin and Louisa Rosenthal, "The Positive Effects of Combined Breathing Techniques and Cold Exposure on Perceived Stress: A Randomised Trial," *Current Psychology* 42, no. 31 (October 7, 2022): 27058–70, https://doi.org/10.1007/s12144-022-03739-y.

29   lowered stress levels: Elissa Epel, PhD, *The Stress Prescription: Seven Days to More Joy and Ease* (New York: Penguin, 2022).

30   the body experiences: Jonathan M. Peake, James F. Markworth, Kazunori Nosaka, Truls Raastad, Glenn D. Wadley, and Vernon G. Coffey, "Modulating Exercise-Induced Hormesis: Does Less Equal More?" *Journal of Applied Psychology* 119, no. 3 (2015): 172–89, https://doi.org/10.1152/japplphysiol.01055.2014.

31   physical and mental benefits: Brianna Chu, Komal Marwaha, Terrence Sanvictores, Ayoola O. Awosika, and Derek Ayers, "Physiology, Stress Reaction," *StatPearls*, May 7, 2024.

32   increasing our stress resilience: Epel, *The Stress Prescription*.

CHAPTER 3: GO WITH THE FLOW: THE ENDOCRINE SYSTEM AND HORMONAL BALANCE

34 regulating functions: "Endocrine System," Cleveland Clinic, November 27, 2019, https://my.clevelandclinic.org/health/body/21201-endocrine -system.

36 or "love drug": Howard E. LeWine, MD, "Oxtytocin: The Love Hormone," Harvard Health Publishing: Harvard Medical School, June 13, 2023, https://www.health.harvard.edu/mind-and-mood/oxytocin-the-love -hormone.

36 *The Hormone Cure*: Sara Gottfried, *The Hormone Cure: Reclaim Balance, Sleep, Sex Drive and Vitality Naturally with the Gottfried Protocol* (New York: Simon & Schuster, 2014).

36 mice lacking dopamine: Richard D. Palmiter, "Dopamine Signaling in the Dorsal Striatum Is Essential for Motivated Behaviors: Lessons from Dopamine-Deficient Mice," *Annals of the New York Academy of Sciences* 1129 (2008): 35–46, https://doi.org/10.1196/annals.1417.003.

40 female brain changes dramatically: Sanjay Mishra, "The Menstrual Cycle Can Reshape Your Brain," *Premium*, October 16, 2024, https://www .nationalgeographic.com/premium/article/menstruation-brain-women -reshape.

42 medical help for them: Ellen B. Gold, Craig Wells, and Marianne O'Neill Rasor, "The Association of Inflammation with Premenstrual Symptoms," *Journal of Women's Health* 25, no. 9 (September 2016): 865–74, https:// doi.org/10.1089/jwh.2015.5529.

42 symptom of hormone imbalance: "What Are Menstrual Irregularities?" NIH, n.d., https://www.nichd.nih.gov/health/topics/menstruation/conditioninfo /irregularities.

42 "onset of menarche": Mengnan Lu, Ruoyang Feng, Yujie Qin, Hongyang Deng, Biyao Lian, Chunyan Yin, and Yanfeng Xiao, "Identifying Envi-ronmental Endocrine Disruptors Associated with the Age at Menarche by Integrating a Transcriptome-Wide Association Study with Chemical-Gene-Interaction Analysis," *Frontiers in Endocrinology* 13 (February 24, 2022): 836527, https://doi.org/10.3389/fendo.2022.836527.

42 have painful cramps: Mark E. Schoep, Theodoor E. Nieboer, Moniek van der Zanden, Did D. M. Braat, and Annemiek W. Nap, "The Impact of Menstrual Symptoms on Everyday Life: A Survey Among 42,879 Women," *American Journal of Obstetrics and Gynecology* 220, no. 6 (2019): 569.e1–e7, https://doi.org/10.1016/j.ajog.2019.02.048.

42 cannot do regular activities: Pallavi Latthe, Rita Champaneria, and Khalid Khan, "Dysmenorrhea," *American Family Physician* 85, no. 4 (February 15, 2012): 386–87.

43 exacerbate psychiatric disorders: Mary Lee Barron, Louise H. Flick, Cynthia A. Cook, Sharon M. Homan, and Claudia Campbell, "Associations Between Psychiatric Disorders and Menstrual Cycle Characteristics," *Archives of Psychi-atric Nursing* 22, no. 5 (October 2008): 254–65, https://doi.org/10.1016/j .apnu.2007.11.001.

46 Research shows: Salman Assad, Hamza H. Khan, Haider Ghazanfar, Zarak H. Khan, Salman Mansoor, Muhammad A. Rahman, Ghulam H. Khan, Bilal Zafar, Usman Tariq, and Shuja A. Malik, "Role of Sex Hormone Levels and

Psychological Stress in the Pathogenesis of Autoimmune Diseases," *Cureus* 9, no. 6 (June 5, 2017): e1315, https://doi.org/10.7759/cureus.1315.

46   one study notes: Ibid.

46   and even infertility: David Prokai and Sarah L. Berga, "Neuroprotection via Reduction in Stress: Altered Menstrual Patterns as a Marker for Stress and Implications for Long-Term Neurologic Health in Women," *International Journal of Molecular Sciences* 17, no. 12 (December 20, 2016): 2147, https://doi.org/10.3390/ijms17122147.

46   to be infertile: Kristin L. Rooney and Alice D. Domar, "The Relationship Between Stress and Infertility," *Dialogues in Clinical Neuroscience* 20, no. 1 (March 2018): 41–47, https://doi.org/10.31887/DCNS.2018.20.1/klrooney.

46   of one study: J. Garcia-Leme and S. P. Farsky, "Hormonal Control of Inflammatory Responses," *Mediators of Inflammation* 2, no. 3 (1993): 181–98, https://doi.org/10.1155/S0962935193000250.

47   in most PMS symptoms: Gold et al., "The Association of Inflammation with Premenstrual Symptoms."

47   to PMS and PMDD: Lara Tiranini and Rossella E. Nappi, "Recent Advances in Understanding/Management of Premenstrual Dysphoric Disorder/Premenstrual Syndrome," *Faculty Reviews* 11 (April 28, 2022): 11, https://doi.org/10.12703/r/11-11.

47   and prostaglandin concentrations: Archana Nagaraja, "Figure 1: Chronic Stress Increases Levels of Prostaglandins," ResearchGate, n.d., https://www.researchgate.net/figure/Chronic-stress-increases-levels-of-prostaglandins-a-Primary-ovarian-tumors-were_fig3_280909179.

48   *The Telomere Effect*: Blackburn and Epel, *The Telomere Effect*.

48   is produced: Jean-Baptiste Bouillon-Minois, Marion Trousselard, David Thivel, Brett Ashley Gordon, Jeannot Schmidt, Farès Moustafa, Charlotte Oris, and Frédéric Dutheil, "Ghrelin as a Biomarker of Stress: A Systematic Review and Meta-Analysis," *Nutrients* 13, no. 3 (February 27, 2021): 784, https://doi.org/10.3390/nu13030784.

48   low-grade inflammation: Sara Castro-Barquero, Rosa Casas, Eric B. Rimm, Anna Tresserra-Rimbau, Dora Romaguera, J. Alfredo Martínez, Jordi Salas-Salvadó, et al., "Loss of Visceral Fat Is Associated with a Reduction in Inflammatory Status in Patients with Metabolic Syndrome," *Molecular Nutrition & Food Research* 67, no. 4 (January 24, 2023): 2200264, https://doi.org/10.1002/mnfr.202200264.

49   production of certain hormones: National Institute of Environmental Health Sciences, "Endocrine Disruptors," n.d., https://www.niehs.nih.gov/health/topics/agents/endocrine.

49   levels of estrogen in women: Luisa María Sánchez-Zamorano, Lourdes Flores-Luna, Angélica Angeles-Lleranes, Carolina Ortega-Olvera, Eduardo Lazcano-Ponce, Isabelle Romieu, Fernando Mainero-Ratchelous, and Gabriela Torres-Mejía, "The Western Dietary Pattern Is Associated with Increased Serum Concentrations of Free Estradiol in Postmenopausal Women: Implications for Breast Cancer Prevention," *Nutrition Research* 36, no. 8 (August 2016): 845–54, https://doi.org/10.1016/j.nutres.2016.04.008.

49   testosterone in men: Tzu-Yu Hu, Yi Chun Chen, Pei Lin, Chun-Kuang Shih, Chyi-Huey Bai, Kuo-Ching Yuan, Shin-Yng Lee, and Jung-Su Chang, "Testosterone-Associated Dietary Pattern Predicts Low Testosterone Levels and Hypogonadism," *Nutrients* 10, no. 11 (November 16, 2018): 1786, https://doi.org/10.3390/nu10111786.

49   insulin and cortisol imbalance: Joseph A. M. J. L. Janssen, "The Impact of Westernization on the Insulin/IGF-I Signaling Pathway and the Metabolic Syndrome: It Is Time for Change," *International Journal of Molecular Sciences* 24, no. 5 (February 25, 2023): 4551, https://doi.org/10.3390/ijms24054551.

50   of some cancers: Jennie L. Lovett, Margo A. Chima, Juliana K. Wexler, Kendall J. Arslanian, Andrea B. Friedman, Chantal B. Yousif, and Beverly I. Strassmann, "Oral Contraceptives Cause Evolutionarily Novel Increases in Hormone Exposure: A Risk Factor for Breast Cancer," *Evolution, Medicine, and Public Health* 2017, no. 1 (June 5, 2017): 97–108, https://doi.org/10.1093/emph/eox009.

50   female stress response: Summer Mengelkoch, Jeffrey Gassen, George M. Slavich, and Sarah E. Hill, "Hormonal Contraceptive Use Is Associated with Differences in Women's Inflammatory and Psychological Reactivity to an Acute Social Stressor," *Brain, Behavior, and Immunity* 115 (January 2024): 747–57, https://doi.org/10.1016/j.bbi.2023.10.033.

52   "adaptability of the hormonal system": Touskova et al., "A Novel Wim Hof Psychophysiological Training Program to Reduce Stress Responses During an Antarctic Expedition."

CHAPTER 4: THE CHEMISTRY BETWEEN WOMEN AND ICE

54   act as an insulating layer: John R. Speakman, "Obesity and Thermoregulation," *Handbook of Clinical Neurology* 156 (2018): 431–43, https://doi.org/10.1016/B978-0-444-63912-7.00026-6.

59   degrees or lower: Wouter D. van Marken Lichtenbelt, Joost W. Vanhommerig, Nanda M. Smulders, Jamie M. A. F. L. Drossaerts, Gerrit J. Kemerink, Nicole D. Bouvy, Patrick Schrauwen, and G. J. Jaap Teule, "Cold-Activated Brown Adipose Tissue in Healthy Men," *New England Journal of Medicine* 360, no. 15 (April 9, 2009): 1500–08, https://doi.org/10.1056/NEJMoa0808718.

60   grams of brown fat: Aaron M. Cypess et al., "Identification and Importance of Brown Adipose Tissue in Adult Humans," *New England Journal of Medicine* (April 9, 2009): 1509–17, https://www.nejm.org/doi/full/10.1056/NEJMoa0810780.

60   white fat into brown fat: Paul Lee, Sheila Smith, Joyce Linderman, Amber B. Courville, Robert J. Brychta, William Dieckmann, Charlotte D. Werner, Kong Y. Chen, and Francesco S. Celi, "Temperature-Acclimated Brown Adipose Tissue Modulates Insulin Sensitivity in Humans," *Diabetes* 63, no. 11 (November 2014): 3686–98, https://doi.org/10.2337/db14-0513.

62   cold water exposure: Kox et al., "The Influence of Concentration/Meditation on Autonomic Nervous System Activity and the Innate Immune Response: A Case Study."

62   Radboud University: Ibid.

62   more body heat: Maarten J. Vosselman, Guy H. E. J. Vijgen, Boris R. M. Kingma, Boudewijn Brans, and Wouter D. van Marken Lichtenbelt, "Frequent Extreme Cold Exposure and Brown Fat and Cold-Induced Thermogenesis: A Study in a Monozygotic Twin," *PLOS ONE* 9, no. 7 (July 11, 2014): e101653, https://doi.org/10.1371/journal.pone.0101653.

62   Michigan study in 2018: Otto Muzik, Kaice T. Reilly, and Vaibhav A. Diwadkar, "'Brain over Body'—A Study on the Willful Regulation of Autonomic Function During Cold Exposure," *NeuroImage* 172 (May 15, 2018): 632–41, https://doi.org/10.1016/j.neuroimage.2018.01.067.

64   clear preference: Thomas Houtermans, Esther K. J. Spetter, Benicio N. Freire, and Paul Smeets, "Stress-Like Glucocorticoid Levels Increase Fasting Hunger and Decrease Resting Energy Expenditure in Humans," *Neuroscience* 394 (2018): 33–44, https://doi.org/10.1016/j.neuroscience.2018.10.018.

64   sensitive in women than men: Matthijs L. Noordzij, Nicholas S. Holmes, Christina N. Murray, Anthony K. Seth, and Robert W. Kentridge, "Distinguishing Between the Metabolic and Hedonic Components of Food Intake: Implications for the Brain Reward System," *Physiology & Behavior* 151 (2015): 377–83, https://doi.org/10.1016/j.physbeh.2015.07.021.

64   study interviewed women: Roxanne N. Felig et al., "When Looking 'Hot' Means Not Feeling Cold: Evidence That Self-Objectification Inhibits Feelings of Being Cold," *British Journal of Social Psychology* 61, no. 2 (2022): 455–70, doi:10.1111/bjso.12489.

65   study by Dutch scientists: Boris Kingma and Wouter van Marken Lichtenbelt, "Energy Consumption in Buildings and Female Thermal Demand," *Nature Climate Change* 5, no. 12 (August 3, 2015): 1054–56, https://doi.org/10.1038/nclimate2741.

65   clear gender inequality: Thomas Parkinson, Stefano Schiavon, Richard de Dear, and Gail Brager, "Overcooling of Offices Reveals Gender Inequity in Thermal Comfort," *Scientific Reports* 11, no. 1 (December 8, 2021): 1–7, https://doi.org/10.1038/s41598-021-03121-1.

65   "dominate in most households": Nicole D. Sintov, Lee V. White, and Hugh Walpole, "Thermostat Wars? The Roles of Gender and Thermal Comfort Negotiations in Household Energy Use Behavior," *PLOS ONE* 14, no. 11 (November 13, 2019): https://doi.org/10.1371/journal.pone.0224198.

65   filled with cold water: Kasiphak Kaikaew, Johanna C. van den Beukel, Sebastian J. C. M. M. Neggers, Axel P. N. Themmen, Jenny A. Visser, and Aldo Grefhorst, "Sex Difference in Cold Perception and Shivering Onset upon Gradual Cold Exposure," *Journal of Thermal Biology* 77 (October 2018): 137–44, https://doi.org/10.1016/j.jtherbio.2018.08.016.

66   brown fat than men: Kasiphak Kaikaew, Aldo Grefhorst, and Jenny A. Visser, "Sex Differences in Brown Adipose Tissue Function: Sex Hormones, Glucocorticoids, and Their Crosstalk," *Frontiers in Endocrinology* 12 (April 13, 2021): 652444, https://doi.org/10.3389/fendo.2021.652444.

68   efficacy with perfect use: Contraceptive Technology, "I-Xlii 1-1006 PART2.pdf," *Contraceptive Efficacy*, n.d., accessed October 16, 2024.

68   raises body temperature: Fiona C. Baker, Duncan Mitchell, and Helen S. Driver, "Oral Contraceptives Alter Sleep and Raise Body Temperature

in Young Women," *Pflügers Archiv* 442, no. 5 (n.d.): 729–37, https://doi.org/10.1007/s004240100582.

74   twelve weeks of cold exposure: Tiina Maria Ikäheimo, Matti Mäntysaari, Tiina Pääkkönen, and Hannu Rintamäki, "Autonomic Nervous Function During Whole-Body Cold Exposure Before and After Cold Acclimation," *Aviation Space and Environmental Medicine* 79, no. 9 (October 2008): 875–82, https://www.researchgate.net/publication/23252519_Autonomic _Nervous_Function_During_Whole-Body_Cold_Exposure_Before_and _After_Cold_Acclimation.

74   over ten days: Ikäheimo et al., "Autonomic Nervous Function During Whole-Body Cold Exposure Before and After Cold Acclimation."

74   cold adaptation disappeared: Joo-Young Lee and Hyo Hyum Lee, "Korean Women Divers 'Haenyeo': Bathing Suits and Acclimatization to Cold," *Journal of the Human-Environment System* 17, no. 1 (December 2014): 1–11, https://www.researchgate.net/publication/286076716_Korean_Women _Divers_'Haenyeo'_Bathing_Suits_and_Acclimatization_to_Cold.

75   cold just the same: Wouter van Marken Lichtenbelt, *Van Rillen Tot Zweten: De Wetenschap Achter Lichaamstemperatuur van Mens En Dier* (Netherlands: New Scientist, 2023).

76   greater than that of air: John W. Castellani and Andrew J. Young, "Human Physiological Responses to Cold Exposure: Acute Responses and Acclimatization to Prolonged Exposure," *Autonomic Neuroscience: Basic & Clinical* 196 (April 2016): 63–74, https://doi.org/10.1016/j.autneu.2016.02.009.

78   charging the object: Gerald H. Pollack, *The Fourth Phase of Water: Beyond Solid, Liquid, and Vapor* (Seattle: Ebner and Sons, 2013).

CHAPTER 5: A DEEP EXHALE: WOMEN AND BREATH

89   fatigue than men: Glenn R. Wylie, Amanda J. Pra Sisto, Helen M. Genova, and John DeLuca, "Frontiers," *Frontiers in Human Neuroscience* 16 (May 8, 2022), https://doi.org/10.3389/fnhum.2022.790006.

89   back to glucose: Jelle Zwaag, Rob ter Horst, Ivana Blaženović, Daniel Stoessel, Jacqueline Ratter, Josephine M. Worseck, Nicolas Schauer, et al., "Involvement of Lactate and Pyruvate in the Anti-Inflammatory Effects Exerted by Voluntary Activation of the Sympathetic Nervous System," *Metabolites* 10, no. 4 (April 10, 2020): 148, https://doi.org/10.3390/metabo10040148.

93   our vagus nerve: Eddie Weitzberg and Jon O. N. Lundberg, "Humming Greatly Increases Nasal Nitric Oxide," *American Journal of Respiratory and Critical Care Medicine* 166, no. 2 (July 15, 2002): 144–45, https://doi.org/10.1164/rccm.200202-138BC.

93   fifteen- to twentyfold: J. O. Lundberg and E. Weitzberg, "Nasal Nitric Oxide in Man," *Thorax* 54, no. 10 (October 1999): 947–52, https://doi.org/10.1136/thx.54.10.947.

94   more oxygen in: Maurice H. Cottle, "The Work, Ways, and Patterns of Nasal Breathing," Presented at American Rhinologic Society Seminar, September 9, 1972.

96   move less air: Antonella LoMauro and Andrea Aliverti, "Sex Differences in Respiratory Function," *Breathe* 14, no. 2 (June 2018): 131–40, https://doi.org/10.1183/20734735.000318.

96 lung capacity than men: Ibid.

96 smaller and rounder: Ibid.

97 one in three women: UCLA Health, "Pelvic Floor Disorders," accessed October 16, 2024, https://www.uclahealth.org/medical-services/womens -pelvic-health/patient-education/pelvic-floor-disorders.

98 breathing difficulties: Courtney Denise Townsel, Sawyer F. Emmer, Winston A. Campbell, and Naveed Hussain, "Gender Differences in Respiratory Morbidity and Mortality of Preterm Neonates," *Frontiers in Pediatrics* 5 (January 30, 2017): 6, https://doi.org/10.3389/fped.2017.00006.

98 of chronic hyperventilation: Helmut W. Ott, Verena Mattle, Ulrich S. Zimmermann, Peter Licht, Kay Moeller, and Ludwig Wildt, "Symptoms of Premenstrual Syndrome May Be Caused by Hyperventilation," *Fertility and Sterility* 86, no. 4 (October 2006): 1001.e17–19, https://doi.org/10.1016/j .fertnstert.2006.01.062.

98 is in her cycle: Ferenc Macsali, Cecilie Svanes, Robert B. Sothern, Bryndis Benediktsdottir, Line Bjørge, Julia Dratva, Karl A. Franklin, et al., "Menstrual Cycle and Respiratory Symptoms in a General Nordic–Baltic Population," *American Journal of Respiratory and Critical Care Medicine* 187, no. 4 (February 15, 2013): 366–73, https://doi.org/10.1164/rccm.201206-1112oc.

103 2–4 percent: Kox et al., "The Influence of Concentration/Meditation on Autonomic Nervous System Activity and the Innate Immune Response."

104 intermittent hypoxia training: Won-Sang Jung, Sung-Woo Kim, and Hun-Young Park, "Interval Hypoxic Training Enhances Athletic Performance and Does Not Adversely Affect Immune Function in Middle- and Long-Distance Runners," *International Journal of Environmental Research and Public Health* 17, no. 6 (March 16, 2020): 1934, https://doi.org/10.3390 /ijerph17061934.

104 levels of erythropoietin: Jung et al., "Interval Hypoxic Training Enhances Athletic Performance and Does Not Adversely Affect Immune Function in Middle- and Long-Distance Runners."

105 in our moms' bellies: Sally L. Dunwoodie, "The Role of Hypoxia in Development of the Mammalian Embryo," *Developmental Cell* 17, no. 6 (December 2009): 755–73, https://doi.org/10.1016/j.devcel.2009.11.008.

106 in a letter: Geert A. Buijze, PhdD, and Maria T. Hopman, PhD, "Controlled Hyperventilation After Training May Accelerate Altitude Acclimatization," *Wilderness & Environmental Medicine* 25, no. 4 (December 2014): 484–86, https://doi.org/10.1016/j.wem.2014.04.009.

107 In one study: Ibid.

107 pelvic floor muscles: Nevin Toprak, San Selva, and Berrak Varhan, "The Role of Diaphragmatic Breathing Exercise on Urinary Incontinence Treatment: A Pilot Study," *Journal of Bodywork and Movement Therapies* 29 (January 2022): 146–53, https://doi.org/10.1016/j.jbmt.2021.10.002.

107 published in 2023: Sonja de Groot, Frank W. L. Ettema, Christel M. C. van Leeuwen, Wendy J. Achterberg, Thomas W. J. Janssen, and Sven P. Hoekstra, "The Effect of Mindset and Breathing Exercises on Physical and Mental Health in Persons with Spinal Cord Injury—A Pilot Feasibility Study," *International Journal of Environmental Research and Public Health* 20, no. 18 (September 20, 2023), https://doi.org/10.3390/ijerph20186784.

108   neutralize the acids: Joseph Pizzorno, "Acidosis: An Old Idea Validated by New Research," *Integrative Medicine* 14, no. 1 (February 2015): 8–12.

108   body's alkaline reserve: Deanna M. Minich and Jeffrey S. Bland, "Acid-Alkaline Balance: Role in Chronic Disease and Detoxification," *Alternative Therapies in Health and Medicine* 13, no. 4 (2007): 62–65.

109   four to five times: Lauren N. Telano and Stephen Baker, "Physiology, Cerebral Spinal Fluid," *StatPearls*, July 4, 2023.

109   products in the brain: Jost M. Kollmeier, Lukas Gürbüz-Reiss, Prativa Sahoo, Simon Badura, Ben Ellebracht, Mathilda Keck, Jutta Gärtner, Hans-Christoph Ludwig, Jens Frahm, and Steffi Dreha-Kulaczewski, "Deep Breathing Couples CSF and Venous Flow Dynamics," *Scientific Reports* 12, no. 1 (February 16, 2022): 1–13, https://doi.org/10.1038/s41598-022-06361-x.

111   Michigan in 2018: Muzik et al., "'Brain over Body'—A Study on the Willful Regulation of Autonomic Function During Cold Exposure."

113   near-death experiences: Rick Strassman, *DMT: The Spirit Molecule: A Doctor's Revolutionary Research into the Biology of Near-Death and Mystical Experiences* (New York: Simon & Schuster, 2000).

114   First, a word of caution: "Breathing Exercises," Wim Hof Method, https://www.wimhofmethod.com/breathing-exercises.

CHAPTER 6: MINDSET: FROM WORRIER TO WARRIOR

122   performed on women: Mishra, "The Menstrual Cycle Can Reshape Your Brain."

122   of the female brain: Paula M. Di Noto, Leorra Newman, Shelley Wall, and Gillian Einstein, "The *Her*munculus: What Is Known About the Representation of the Female Body in the Brain?" *Cerebral Cortex* 23, no. 5 (April 17, 2012): 1005–13, https://doi.org/10.1093/cercor/bhs005.

123   get ahead of the game: Radu Predoiu, Alexandra Predoiu, Georgeta Mitrache, and Madalina Firanescu, "Visualisation Techniques in Sport – the Mental Road Map for Success," *Discobolul – Physical Education, Sport and Kinetotherapy Journal* 59, no. 3 (September 2020): 245–56.

123   working in hotel housekeeping: Alia J. Crum and Ellen J. Langer, "Mind-Set Matters," *Psychological Science* 18, no. 2 (February 2007): 165–71, https://doi.org/10.1111/j.1467-9280.2007.01867.x.

124   pain as morphine: Jon D. Levine, Newton C. Gordon, Richard Smith, and Howard L. Fields, "Analgesic Responses to Morphine and Placebo in Individuals with Postoperative Pain," *Pain* 10, no. 3 (June 1981): 379–89, https://doi.org/10.1016/0304-3959(81)90099-3.

124   completely benign substance: Ulrike Bingel, Vishvarani Wanigasekera, Katja Wiech, Roisin Ni Mhuircheartaigh, Michael C. Lee, Markus Ploner, and Irene Tracey, "The Effect of Treatment Expectation on Drug Efficacy: Imaging the Analgesic Benefit of the Opioid Remifentanil," *Science Translational Medicine* 3, no. 70 (February 16, 2011), https://doi.org/10.1126/scitranslmed.3001244.

125   more connectivity and activity: Bronte Ficek-Tani, Corey Horien, Suyeon Ju, Wanwan Xu, Nancy Li, Cheryl Lacadie, Xilin Shen, Dustin Scheinost, Todd Constable, and Carolyn Fredericks, "Sex Differences in Default Mode Network Connectivity in Healthy Aging Adults," *Cerebral Cortex* 33, no. 10 (May 9, 2023): 6139–51, https://doi.org/10.1093/cercor/bhac491.

126   contributor to breast cancer: Gabor Maté, *When the Body Says No: Under-standing the Stress-Disease Connection* (New York: John Wiley & Sons, 2011).

126   twice as likely: Remes et al., "A Systematic Review of Reviews on the Prevalence of Anxiety Disorders in Adult Populations."

127   *Barbie* movie: *Barbie*, Warner Bros., 2023.

129   half their time: Matthew A. Killingsworth and Daniel T. Gilbert, "A Wandering Mind Is an Unhappy Mind," *Science* 330, no. 6006 (November 12, 2010): 932, https://doi.org/10.1126/science.1192439.

131   measured in brain scans: Muzik et al., "The Impact of a Focused Behavioral Intervention on Brain Cannabinoid Signaling and Interoceptive Function: Implications for Mood and Anxiety."

131   thoughts and feelings: Omar Almahayni and Lucy Hammond, "Does the Wim Hof Method Have a Beneficial Impact on Physiological and Psychological Outcomes in Healthy and Non-Healthy Participants? A Systematic Review," Cold Spring Harbor Laboratory, May 29, 2023, http://dx.doi.org/10.1101/2023.05.28.23290653.

131   woman's brain changes: Mishra, "The Menstrual Cycle Can Reshape Your Brain."

134   types of future stressors: Muzik et al., "The Impact of a Focused Behavioral Intervention on Brain Cannabinoid Signaling and Interoceptive Function: Implications for Mood and Anxiety."

134   compared a group: Epel, *The Stress Prescription*.

CHAPTER 7: THE WHM FOR PREGNANCY, POSTPARTUM, AND MENOPAUSE

139   thirty years old: Centraal Bureau voor de Statistiek, "Kinderen Krijgen," accessed October 21, 2024, https://www.cbs.nl/nl-nl/visualisaties/dashboard-bevolking/levensloop/kinderen-krijgen.

139   morning cortisol levels: Bheena Vyshali Karunyam, Abdul Kadir Abdul Karim, Isa Naina Mohamed, Azizah Ugusman, Wael Mohamed, Mohd Faizal Ahmad, Muhammad Azrai Abu, and Jaya Kumar, "Infertility and Cortisol: A Systematic Review," *Frontiers*, June 29, 2023, https://www.researchgate.net/publication/372411103_Infertility_and_cortisol_a_systematic_review.

139   Additionally, inflammation: Oluwafemi Adeleke Ojo, Pearl Ifunanya Nwafor-Ezeh, Damilare Emmanuel Rotimi, Matthew Iyobhebhe, Akingbolabo Daniel Ogunlakin, and Adebola Busola Ojo, "Apoptosis, Inflammation, and Oxidative Stress in Infertility: A Mini Review," *Toxicology Reports* 10 (2023): 448–62, https://doi.org/10.1016/j.toxrep.2023.04.006.

141   "risk to the fetus": Robert G. McMurray and Vern L. Katz, "Thermoregulation in Pregnancy," *Sports Medicine* 10, no. 3 (November 25, 2012): 146–58, https://doi.org/10.2165/00007256-199010030-00002.

141   regarding heat exposure: Nicholas Ravanelli, William Casasola, Timothy English, Kate M. Edwards, and Ollie Jay, "Heat Stress and Fetal Risk. Environmental Limits for Exercise and Passive Heat Stress During Pregnancy: A Systematic Review with Best Evidence Synthesis," *British Journal of Sports Medicine* 53, no. 13 (2019): 799–805, doi:10.1136/bjsports-2017-097914.

142   nonpregnant women showed: Megan Pound, Heather Massey, Sasha Roseneil, Ruth Williamson, C. Mark Harper, Mike Tipton, Jill Shawe,

Malika Felton, and Joyce C. Harper, "How Do Women Feel Cold Water Swimming Affects Their Menstrual and Perimenopausal Symptoms?" *Post Reproductive Health* 30, no. 1 (January 25, 2024): 11–27, https://doi .org/10.1177/20533691241227100.

142 improved birth outcomes: Leo Gundle and Amelia Atkinson, "Pregnancy, Cold Water Swimming and Cortisol: The Effect of Cold Water Swimming on Obstetric Outcomes," *Medical Hypotheses* 144 (November 2020): 109977, https://doi.org/10.1016/j.mehy.2020.109977.

142 increase insulin sensitivity: Ibid.

144 50 percent of women: Kripa Balaram and Raman Marwaha, "Postpartum Blues," *StatPearls*, March 6, 2023.

147 on menopause: Kimberly Peacock, Karen Carlson, and Kari M. Ketvertis, "Menopause," *StatPearls*, December 21, 2023.

148 last fifty years: Kerstin Rödström, Lilian Weman, Valter Sundh, and Cecilia Björkelund, "Perception of Higher Frequency of Daily Hot Flashes in 50-Year-Old Women Today: A Study of Trends over Time During 48 Years in the Population Study of Women in Gothenburg, Sweden," *Menopause* 29, no. 10 (October 1, 2022): 1124–29, https://doi.org/10.1097 /GME.0000000000002033.

149 severe menopause symptoms: Megan Arnot, Emily H. Emmott, and Ruth Mace, "The Relationship Between Social Support, Stressful Events, and Menopause Symptoms." *PLOS ONE* 16, no. 1 (January 27, 2021): e0245444, https://doi.org/10.1371/journal.pone.0245444.

149 and inflammation levels: Andrei Mihai Malutan, Mihu Dan, Costin Nicolae, and Mihu Carmen, "Proinflammatory and Anti-Inflammatory Cytokine Changes Related to Menopause," *Przeglad Menopauzalny = Menopause Review* 13, no. 3 (June 2014): 162–68, https://doi.org/10.5114 /pm.2014.43818.

149 "systemic inflammatory phase": Micheline McCarthy and Ami P. Raval, "The Peri-Menopause in a Woman's Life: A Systemic Inflammatory Phase That Enables Later Neurodegenerative Disease," *Journal of Neuroinflammation* 17, no. 1 (October 23, 2020): 1–14, https://doi.org/10.1186 /s12974-020-01998-9.

149 influenced by estrogen: Gengfan Liang, Audrey Siew Foong Kow, Rohana Yusof, Chau Ling Tham, Yu-Cheng Ho, and Ming Tatt Lee, "Menopause-Associated Depression: Impact of Oxidative Stress and Neuroinflammation on the Central Nervous System—A Review," *Biomedicines* 12, no. 1 (January 15, 2024): 184, https://doi.org/10.3390/biomedicines12010184.

149 in mental health: Ibid.

150 published in 2024: Pound et al., "How Do Women Feel Cold Water Swimming Affects Their Menstrual and Perimenopausal Symptoms?"

150 menopause-related burnout: Lesley Salem, "Why Businesses Should Be More Aware of Menopause-Related Burnout," *PeopleManagement*, February 7, 2022, https://www.peoplemanagement.co.uk/article /1742024/why-businesses-should-be-more-aware-of-menopause-related -burnout.

151 in one study: P. Srámek, M. Simecková, L. Janský, J. Savlíková, and S. Vybíral, "Human Physiological Responses to Immersion into Water of Different

Temperatures," *European Journal of Applied Physiology* 81, no. 5 (March 2000): 436–42, https://doi.org/10.1007/s004210050065.

151   report hot flashes: Ellen W. Freeman, Mary D. Sammel, Hui Lin, Clarisa R. Gracia, Shiv Kapoor, and Tahmina Ferdousi, "The Role of Anxiety and Hormonal Changes in Menopausal Hot Flashes," *Menopause* 12, no. 3 (2005): 258–66, https://doi.org/10.1097/01.gme.0000142440 .49698.b7.

151   clinical trial: Richa Sood, Amit Sood, Sherry L. Wolf, Breanna M. Linquist, Heshan Liu, Jeff A. Sloan, Daniel V. Satele, Charles L. Loprinzi, and Debra L. Barton, "Paced Breathing Compared with Usual Breathing for Hot Flashes," *Menopause* 20, no. 2 (February 2013): 179–84, https://doi .org/10.1097/gme.0b013e31826934b6.

152   that are common: Ashley Welch, "Menopause and Heart Palpitations: Risks, Symptoms, and Concerns," EverydayHealth, December 22, 2020, https:// www.everydayhealth.com/menopause/menopausal-heart-palpitations-can -cause-distress-may-signal-serious-health-issue/.

152   stress and sleep deprivation: Susan X. Zhao, Hilary A. Tindle, Joseph C. Larson, Nancy F. Woods, Michael H. Crawford, Valerie Hoover, Elena Salmoirago-Blotcher, Aladdin H. Shadyab, Marcia L. Stefanick, and Marco V. Perez, "Association Between Insomnia, Stress Events, and Other Psychosocial Factors and Incident Atrial Fibrillation in Postmenopausal Women: Insights from the Women's Health Initiative," *Journal of the American Heart Association* 12, no. 17 (September 5, 2023), https://doi.org/10.1161/ jaha.123.030030.

153   during these years: R.R. Wing, K. A. Matthews, L. H. Kuller, E. N. Meilahn, and P. L. Plantinga, "Weight Gain at the Time of Menopause," *Archives of Internal Medicine* 151, no. 1 (January 1991): 97–102.

153   acute cold exposure: Chuanyi Huo, Zikai Song, Jianli Yin, Ying Zhu, Xiaohan Miao, Honghao Qian, Jia Wang, Lin Ye, and Liting Zhou, "Effect of Acute Cold Exposure on Energy Metabolism and Activity of Brown Adipose Tissue in Humans: A Systematic Review and Meta-Analysis," *Frontiers in Physiology* 13 (June 28, 2022): 917084, https://doi.org/10.3389/ fphys.2022.917084.

153   increase insulin sensitivity: Yoanna M. Ivanova and Denis P. Blondin, "Examining the Benefits of Cold Exposure as a Therapeutic Strategy for Obesity and Type 2 Diabetes," *Journal of Applied Physiology* 130, no. 5 (May 1, 2021): 1448–59, https://doi.org/10.1152/japplphysiol .00934.2020.

153   insulin sensitivity: Magdalena Gibas-Dorna, Zuzanna Chęcińska, Emilia Korek, Justyna Kupsz, Anna Sowińska, and Hanna Krauss, "Cold Water Swimming Beneficially Modulates Insulin Sensitivity in Middle-Aged Individuals," *Journal of Aging and Physical Activity* 24, no. 4 (October 2016): 547–54, https://doi.org/10.1123/japa.2015-0222.

153   white fat to brown fat: Paul Lee, Joyce D. Linderman, Sheila Smith, Robert J. Brychta, Juan Wang, Christopher Idelson, Rachel M. Perron, et al., "Irisin and FGF21 Are Cold-Induced Endocrine Activators of Brown Fat Function in Humans," *Cell Metabolism* 19, no. 2 (February 4, 2014): 302–9, https:// doi.org/10.1016/j.cmet.2013.12.017.

CHAPTER 8: THE WHM FOR INFLAMMATORY AND AUTOIMMUNE DISEASE

154   more than one: Peter Boersma, "Prevalence of Multiple Chronic Conditions Among US Adults, 2018," *Preventing Chronic Disease* 17 (September 18, 2020), https://doi.org/10.5888/pcd17.200130.

155   results even show: Hemmo A. Drexhage, *Immuno-Psychiatrie: Het Immuunsysteem Uit Balans Als Oorzaak van Psychiatrische Aandoeningen* (Amsterdam: SWP Publishing, 2023).

155   mortality worldwide: David Furman, Judith Campisi, Eric Verdin, Pedro Carrera-Bastos, Sasha Targ, Claudio Franceschi, Luigi Ferrucci, et al., "Chronic Inflammation in the Etiology of Disease Across the Life Span," *Nature Medicine* 25, no. 12 (December 5, 2019): 1822–32, https://doi.org/10.1038/s41591-019-0675-0.

155   people die: Roma Pahwa, Amandeep Goyal, and Ishwarlal Jialal, "Chronic Inflammation," *StatPearls*, August 7, 2023.

155   prescribed medication: Peter C. Gøtzsche, "Our Prescription Drugs Kill Us in Large Numbers," *Polskie Archiwum Medycyny Wewnetrznej* 124, no. 11 (2014): 628–34, https://doi.org/10.20452/pamw.2503.

156   weigh about 2.6 pounds: Ron Sender, Yarden Weiss, Yoav Navon, Idan Milo, Nofar Azulay, Leeat Keren, Shai Fuchs, Danny Ben-Zvi, Elad Noor, and Ron Milo, "The Total Mass, Number, and Distribution of Immune Cells in the Human Body," *Proceedings of the National Academy of Sciences* 120, no. 44 (October 23, 2023), https://doi.org/10.1073/pnas.2308511120.

158   increased auto-antibodies: Vanessa L. Kronzer, Stanley Louis Bridges Jr., and John M. Davis III, "Why Women Have More Autoimmune Diseases Than Men: An Evolutionary Perspective," *Evolutionary Applications* 14, no. 3 (December 1, 2020): 629–33, https://doi.org/10.1111/eva.13167.

158   postpartum and in perimenopause: Fariha Angum, Tahir Khan, Jasndeep Kaler, Lena Siddiqui, and Azhar Hussain, "The Prevalence of Autoimmune Disorders in Women: A Narrative Review," *Cureus* 12, no. 5 (May 13, 2020): e8094, https://doi.org/10.7759/cureus.8094.

158   risk equalizes: Max Nieuwdorp, *The Power of Hormones: The New Science of How Hormones Shape Every Aspect of Our Lives* (New York: Simon & Schuster, 2024).

158   Retrospective studies: Assad et al., "Role of Sex Hormone Levels and Psychological Stress in the Pathogenesis of Autoimmune Diseases."

159   Radboud study: Kox et al., "Voluntary Activation of the Sympathetic Nervous System and Attenuation of the Innate Immune Response in Humans."

160   WHM has shown: Ibid.

160   with autoimmune disease: G. A. Buijze, H. M. Y. De Jong, M. Kox, M. G. van de Sande, D. Van Schaardenburg, R. M. Van Vugt, C. D. Popa, P. Pickkers, and D. L. P. Baeten, "An Add-On Training Program Involving Breathing Exercises, Cold Exposure, and Meditation Attenuates Inflammation and Disease Activity in Axial Spondyloarthritis – A Proof of Concept Trial," *PLOS ONE* 14, no. 12 (December 2, 2019): e0225749, https://doi.org/10.1371/journal.pone.0225749.

161   acute mountain sickness: Buijze et al., "Controlled Hyperventilation After Training May Accelerate Altitude Acclimatization."

161   of the population: Alvaro Gonzalez-Cantero, María Magdalena Constantin, Annunziata Dattola, Tom Hillary, Elise Kleyn, and Nina Magnolo, "Gender Perspective in Psoriasis: A Scoping Review and Proposal of Strategies for Improved Clinical Practice by European Dermatologists," *International Journal of Women's Dermatology* 9, no. 4 (November 1, 2023): e112, https://doi.org/10.1097/JW9.0000000000000112.

162   a clinical trial: J. Czarnecki, "Combination of Breathing Exercises, Cold Exposure, and Meditation Mitigate Psoriasis – Open Label, Randomized, Controlled Trial," *Journal of Investigative Dermatology* 141, no. 10 (October 2021): S153, https://doi.org/10.1016/j.jid.2021.08.026.

163   IL-6 and TNF-α: Andrei M. Malutan, Tudor Drugan, Nicolae Costin, Razvan Ciortea, Carmen Bucuri, Maria P. Rada, and Dan Mihu, "Pro-Inflammatory Cytokines for Evaluation of Inflammatory Status in Endometriosis," *Central European Journal of Immunology* 40, no. 1 (2015): 96–102, https://doi.org/10.5114/ceji.2015.50840.

165   8 to 13 percent: "Polycystic Ovary Syndrome (PCOS) – PI Prof. Joop Laven, MD PhD," Erasmus MC, accessed October 23, 2024, https://www.erasmusmc.nl/en/research/groups/polycystic-ovary-syndrome-pcos.

165   PCOS is also linked: Gottfried, *The Hormone Cure*.

166   high cortisol: Barnali Ray Basu, Olivia Chowdhury, and Sudip Kumar Saha, "Possible Link Between Stress-Related Factors and Altered Body Composition in Women with Polycystic Ovarian Syndrome," *Journal of Human Reproductive Sciences* 11, no. 1 (2018): 10–18, https://doi.org/10.4103/jhrs.JHRS_78_17.

166   onset of this condition: Mayo Clinic, "Polycystic Ovary Syndrome (PCOS) – Symptoms and Causes," accessed October 23, 2024, https://www.mayoclinic.org/diseases-conditions/pcos/symptoms-causes/syc-20353439.

166   depression and anxiety: Zoe S. Markomanolaki, Xanthi Tigani, Thomas Siamatras, Flora Bacopoulou, Athanasios Tsartsalis, Artemios Artemiadis, Vasileios Megalooikonomou, Dimitrios Vlachakis, George P. Chrousos, and Christina Darviri, "Stress Management in Women with Hashimoto's Thyroiditis: A Randomized Controlled Trial," *Journal of Molecular Biochemistry* 8, no. 1 (2019): 3–12.

166   more likely: NIH–National Institute of Diabetes and Digestive and Kidney Diseases, "Hashimoto's Disease," November 16, 2022, https://www.niddk.nih.gov/health-information/endocrine-diseases/hashimotos-disease.

167   have chronic pain: S. Michaela Rikard, "Chronic Pain Among Adults— United States, 2019–2021," *MMWR: Morbidity and Mortality Weekly Report* 72 (April 13, 2023), https://doi.org/10.15585/mmwr.mm7215a1.

167   increasing pain tolerance: Jelle Zwaag, Hans Timmerman, Peter Pickkers, and Matthijs Kox, "Modulation of Pain Sensitivity," *Journal of Pain Research* 16 (June 13, 2023): 1979–91, https://doi.org/10.2147/JPR.S400408.

168   and cannabinoids: Muzik et al., "The Impact of a Focused Behavioral Intervention on Brain Cannabinoid Signaling and Interoceptive Function: Implications for Mood and Anxiety."

168   condition are women: Ilga Ruschak, Pilar Montesó-Curto, Lluís Rosselló, Carina Aguilar Martín, Laura Sánchez-Montesó, and Loren Toussaint, "Fibromyalgia Syndrome Pain in Men and Women: A Scoping Review,"

Healthcare 11, no. 2 (January 11, 2023): 223, https://doi.org/10.3390 /healthcare11020223.

168   more severe pain: Ibid.

169   prevention and treatment: Cancer.gov, "Stress and Cancer," accessed October 23, 2024, https://www.cancer.gov/about-cancer/coping/feelings /stress-fact-sheet#can-stress-cause-cancer.

169   glucose starvation: Takahiro Seki, Yunlong Yang, Xiaoting Sun, Sharon Lim, Sisi Xie, Ziheng Guo, Wenjing Xiong, et al., "Brown-Fat-Mediated Tumour Suppression by Cold-Altered Global Metabolism," *Nature* 608, no. 7922 (August 3, 2022): 421–28, https://doi.org/10.1038/s41586 -022-05030-3.

169   a pilot study on: Tatiana P. Grazioso and Nabil Djouder, "A Mechanistic View of the Use of Cold Temperature in the Treatment of Cancer," *iScience* 26, no. 4 (March 30, 2023): 106511, doi:10.1016/j.isci.2023.106511.

171   how interconnected: Drexhage, *Immuno-Psychiatrie*.

CHAPTER 9: THE WHM FOR MENTAL HEALTH

172   compared to men: "Men and Mental Health," National Institute of Mental Health, n.d., https://www.nimh.nih.gov/health/topics/men-and-mental-health.

173   research shows: Ariel B. Handy, Shelly F. Greenfield, Kimberly A. Yonkers, and Laura A. Payne, "Psychiatric Symptoms Across the Menstrual Cycle in Adult Women: A Comprehensive Review," *Harvard Review of Psychiatry* 30, no. 2 (2022): 100–17, https://doi.org/10.1097/HRP.0000000000000329.

174   In one example: Andrea L. Roberts, Tianyi Huang, Karestan C. Koenen, Yongjoo Kim, Laura D. Kubzansky, and Shelley S. Tworoger, "Posttraumatic Stress Disorder Is Associated with Increased Risk of Ovarian Cancer: A Prospective and Retrospective Longitudinal Cohort Study," *Cancer Research* 79, no. 19 (October 1, 2019): 5113–20, https://doi.org/10.1158/0008-5472. CAN-19-1222.

174   "Brain over Body" study: Muzik et al., "'Brain over Body'—A Study on the Willful Regulation of Autonomic Function During Cold Exposure."

175   a retrospective study: James Kennedy and Marc Cohen, "Invitation to Participate in a Research Project," Project Title: "Wim Hof Method Survey," School of Health & Biomedical Sciences, RMIT University, n.d., https:// rmit.au1.qualtrics.com/CP/File.php?F=F_3r6ewWMmL6BiuTb.

176   six-week WHM training: Muzik et al., "The Impact of a Focused Behavioral Intervention on Brain Cannabinoid Signaling and Interoceptive Function: Implications for Mood and Anxiety."

177   called microglial cells: Ibid.

177   in collaboration: Epel, *The Stress Prescription*.

178   adults: Dan Witters, "U.S. Depression Rates Reach New Highs," Gallup, May 17, 2023, https://news.gallup.com/poll/505745/depression-rates -reach-new-highs.aspx.

178   likely to suffer: Kalkidan Hassen Abate, "Gender Disparity in Prevalence of Depression Among Patient Population: A Systematic Review," *Ethiopian Journal of Health Sciences* 23, no. 3 (November 2013): 283–88, https://doi .org/10.4314/ejhs.v23i3.11.

178   a strong link: "Many Mental-Health Conditions Have Bodily Triggers," *The Economist*, April 24, 2024, https://www.economist.com/science-and -technology/2024/04/24/many-mental-health-conditions-have-bodily -triggers.

178   UK Biobank: Ibid.

179   case study: Christoffer van Tulleken, Michael Tipton, Heather Massey, and C. Mark Harper, "Open Water Swimming as a Treatment for Major Depressive Disorder," *BMJ Case Reports* (August 21, 2018): bcr2018225007, https://doi.org/10.1136/bcr-2018-225007.

179   with mild depression: Epel, *The Stress Prescription*.

181   twice as likely: Bradley Olson, "How Anxiety Impacts Men Versus Women," UNC Men's Health Program, August 29, 2019, https://www.med.unc.edu /menshealth/how-anxiety-impacts-men-versus-women/.

181   dramatically increases: "About the CDC-Kaiser ACE Study," CDC, June 3, 2024, https://www.cdc.gov/violenceprevention/aces/about.html.

182   controlled study: Jemma King, "ANZCTR: Effectiveness of Combined Breathwork and Cold Immersion for Psychological and Physiological Measures of Wellbeing and Performance," Registration, n.d., https://www .anzctr.org.au/Trial/Registration/TrialReview.aspx?id=386317.

CHAPTER 10: BIOHACK WITH THE WHM: LONGEVITY AND THE FEMALE CYCLE

185   increased dramatically: "Americans Are Living Longer Than Ever," PRB, accessed October 24, 2024, https://www.prb.org/resources/americans-are -living-longer-than-ever/.

187   of your telomeres: Marlies Schellnegger, Elisabeth Hofmann, Martina Carnieletto, and Lars-Peter Kamolz, "Frontiers," *Frontiers in Aging* 5 (January 24, 2024), https://doi.org/10.3389/fragi.2024.1339317.

187   25 percent determined: "Americans Are Living Longer Than Ever," PRB.

187   Some experts: Dr. Kenneth R. Pelletier, *Change Your Genes, Change Your Life: Creating Optimal Health with the New Science of Epigenetics* (San Rafael, California: Origin Press, 2018): 28–30.

188   cold shock proteins: Riikka Keto-Timonen, Nina Hietala, Eveliina Palonen, Anna Hakakorpi, Miia Lindström, and Hannu Korkeala, "Cold Shock Proteins: A Minireview with Special Emphasis on Csp-Family of Enteropathogenic *Yersinia*," *Frontiers in Microbiology* 7 (July 22, 2016): 1151, https:// doi.org/10.3389/fmicb.2016.01151.

189   muscle mass: Nana Chung, Jonghoon Park, and Kiwon Lim, "The Effects of Exercise and Cold Exposure on Mitochondrial Biogenesis in Skeletal Muscle and White Adipose Tissue," *Journal of Exercise Nutrition & Biochemistry* 21, no. 2 (June 30, 2017): 39–47, https://doi.org/10.20463 /jenb.2017.0020.

189   Neuroprotective properties: Hyun Ju Lee, Hafiza Alirzayeva, Seda Koyuncu, Amirabbas Rueber, Alireza Noormohammadi, and David Vilchez, "Cold Temperature Extends Longevity and Prevents Disease-Related Protein Aggregation Through PA28γ-Induced Proteasomes," *Nature Aging* 3, no. 5 (April 3, 2023): 546–66, https://doi.org/10.1038/s43587-023-00383-4.

189   damaged neurons: Wenlong Xia, Libo Su, and Jianwei Jiao, "Cold-Induced Protein RBM3 Orchestrates Neurogenesis via Modulating Yap mRNA

Stability in Cold Stress," *Journal of Cell Biology* 217, no. 10 (October 1, 2018): 3464–79, https://doi.org/10.1083/jcb.201801143.

189 Enhancing autophagy: Winifred W. Yau, Kiraely Adam Wong, Jin Zhou, Nivetha Kanakaram Thimmukonda, Yajun Wu, Boon-Huat Bay, Brijesh Kumar Singh, and Paul Michael Yen, "Chronic Cold Exposure Induces Autophagy to Promote Fatty Acid Oxidation, Mitochondrial Turnover, and Thermogenesis in Brown Adipose Tissue," *iScience* 24, no. 5 (May 2021): 102434, https://doi.org/10.1016/j.isci.2021.102434.

189 against neurodegeneration: Takuma Aihara, "Cold Shock as a Possible Remedy for Neurodegenerative Disease," *International Journal of Neurology and Neurotherapy* 3, no. 4 (August 31, 2016), https://doi.org/10.23937/2378-3001/3/4/1053.

189 boost neurogeneration: Lee et al., "Cold Temperature Extends Longevity and Prevents Disease-Related Protein Aggregation Through PA28γ-Induced Proteasomes."

189 have also linked: Ying Chen and John Lyga, "Brain-Skin Connection: Stress, Inflammation and Skin Aging," *Inflammation & Allergy Drug Targets* 13, no. 3 (2014): 177–90, https://doi.org/10.2174/1871528113666140522104422.

191 World Health Organization: WHO, "Diabetes," World Health Organization: WHO, April 5, 2023, https://www.who.int/news-room/fact-sheets/detail/diabetes.

191 insulin sensitivity: Mark J. W. Hanssen, Joris Hoeks, Boudewijn Brans, Anouk A. J. J. van der Lans, Gert Schaart, José J. van den Driessche, Johanna A. Jörgensen, et al., "Short-Term Cold Acclimation Improves Insulin Sensitivity in Patients with Type 2 Diabetes Mellitus," *Nature Medicine* 21, no. 8 (August 2015): 863–65, https://doi.org/10.1038/nm.3891.

192 Research shows: Srámek et al., "Human Physiological Responses to Immersion into Water of Different Temperatures."

193 carbon dioxide: James McIntosh, "Majority of Weight Loss Occurs 'via Breathing,'" *Medical News Today*, December 17, 2014, https://www.medicalnewstoday.com/articles/287046.

193 studies showing: Annie Atherton, "The Sleep Gender Gap: Nighttime Disparities Between Women and Men," Sleep Foundation, March 5, 2024, https://www.sleepfoundation.org/sleep-news/the-sleep-gender-gap-nighttime-disparities-between-women-and-men.

193 more likely: Ibid.

193 and depression: "Health Risks of Poor Sleep," Johns Hopkins Medicine, n.d., https://www.hopkinsmedicine.org/health/wellness-and-prevention/health-risks-of-poor-sleep.

193 recent study: H. Li, F. Qian, L. Han, W. Feng, D. Zheng, X. Guo, and H. Zhang, "Association of Healthy Sleep Patterns with Risk of Mortality and Life Expectancy at Age of 30 Years: A Population-Based Cohort Study," *QJM: Monthly Journal of the Association of Physicians* 117, no. 3 (March 27, 2024): 177–86, https://doi.org/10.1093/qjmed/hcad237.

196 more brown fat: Susanna Søberg, Johan Löfgren, Frederik E. Philipsen, Michal Jensen, Adam E. Hansen, Esben Ahrens, Kristin B. Nystrup, et al., "Altered Brown Fat Thermoregulation and Enhanced Cold-Induced Thermogenesis in Young, Healthy, Winter-Swimming Men," *Cell Reports*

Medicine 2, no. 10 (October 11, 2021): 100408, https://doi.org/10.1016/j
.xcrm.2021.100408.

196   ten days: Hanssen et al., "Short-Term Cold Acclimation Improves Insulin
Sensitivity in Patients with Type 2 Diabetes Mellitus."

196   in a study: Nikolai A. Shevchuk, "Adapted Cold Shower as a Potential
Treatment for Depression," *Medical Hypotheses* 70, no. 5 (2008): 995–1001,
https://doi.org/10.1016/j.mehy.2007.04.052.

196   in the Netherlands: Geert A. Buijze, Inger N. Sierevelt, Bas C. J. M. van
der Heijden, Marcel G. Dijkgraaf, and Monique H. W. Frings-Dresen,
"The Effect of Cold Showering on Health and Work: A Randomized Controlled Trial," *PLOS ONE* 11, no. 9 (September 15, 2016), https://doi
.org/10.1371/journal.pone.0161749.

198   with thermoregulation: Dale Brigham, "Iron and Thermoregulation: A Review," *Critical Reviews in Food Science & Nutrition*, December 1, 1996.

200   in the brain: Hadine Joffe, Anouk de Wit, Jamie Coborn, Sybil Crawford,
Marlene Freeman, Aleta Wiley, Geena Athappilly, et al., "Impact of Estradiol
Variability and Progesterone on Mood in Perimenopausal Women with Depressive Symptoms," *Journal of Clinical Endocrinology and Metabolism* 105,
no. 3 (March 1, 2020): dgz181, https://doi.org/10.1210/clinem/dgz181.

CHAPTER 11: BECOMING AN ICEWOMAN

203   stroll in nature: Yasuhiro Kotera, Miles Richardson, and David Sheffield,
"Effects of Shinrin-Yoku (Forest Bathing) and Nature Therapy on Mental
Health: A Systematic Review and Meta-Analysis," *International Journal of
Mental Health and Addiction* 20, no. 1 (July 28, 2020): 337–61, https://doi
.org/10.1007/s11469-020-00363-4.

203   ten-minute walk: EurekAlert!, "Spending Time in Nature Reduces Stress,
Research Finds," n.d., https://www.eurekalert.org/news-releases/921456.

203   50 percent: "How We Proved Two Nights in Nature Improves Wellbeing
and Reduces Burnout," Unyoked, accessed October 24, 2024, https://www
.unyoked.co/Journal/introducing-the-worlds-first-global-nature-study.

215   In one study: Elissa S. Epel, Alexandra D. Crosswell, Stefanie E. Mayer,
Aric A. Prather, George M. Slavich, Eli Puterman, et al., "More Than a
Feeling: A Unified View of Stress Measurement for Population Science,"
Frontiers in Neuroendocrinology 49 (2018): 151, https://doi.org/10.1016/j
.yfrne.2018.03.001.

219   28 percent: Peter M. Gollwitzer, "Implementation Intentions: Strong Effects
of Simple Plans," *American Psychologist* 54, no. 7 (1999): 493–503, https://
doi.org/10.1037//0003-066x.54.7.493.

INDEX

ABOUT THE AUTHORS

ISABELLE HOF, MSc, built and now advises the Wim Hof Method Academy, is cofounder of the Icewomen Community, and is a WHM instructor. She holds an MA in psychology and has been involved with Innerfire BV since its beginnings, including organizing expeditions, creating the instructor video course, and coordinating scientific studies.

LAURA HOF, MA, is a holistic therapist, speaker, facilitator, cofounder of the Icewomen Community, and very active WHM instructor. She has held a number of positions at Innerfire BV and now leads her own travels and co-teaches with Wim. She earned two history master specializations, history of international relations and American studies, and has worked for various international institutions as well.